The Grandma Mediterra

Traditional Recipes for Healthy Eati

Table of Contents

INTRODUCTION

A Mediterranean diet has been praised for providing a wide range of health benefits ranging from reduced risk of cancer to improved heart health. This type of diet has been studied by medical experts and diet professionals. Here are some benefits of a Mediterranean diet that is backed by science:

Increases Life Span and Promotes Heart Health

Mediterranean diet is widely known to have a positive effect on the health of your heart. According to a landmark study, 7,000 people were selected to follow a strict Mediterranean diet that consisted of nuts and olive oil. These people significantly lowered the risk of major cardiovascular events like a stroke or a heart attack. They also had fewer cardiovascular disease risk factors like central obesity.

In food items like fatty fish, olive oil, and nuts, the presence of healthy fats is the key factor that contributes to this fact. For instance, 'bad' LDL cholesterol is lowered by Omega-3 fats; additionally, it also raises the 'good' HDL cholesterol levels, improves insulin resistance, and reduces inflammation. The high levels of antioxidants and fiber from red wine, fruits, and vegetables have a cardio-protective effect as well.

Since you will improve the health of your heart, a Mediterranean diet will also increase your life span.

Promotes Metabolism and Healthy Weight

Mediterranean diets focus on food that is whole and real – particularly those that have high fiber content. This makes the diet a great choice for anyone who is looking to improve their overall metabolic health. According to experts, a Mediterranean diet that contains high-fiber content makes you less likely to gain weight by keeping you full and improving glucose and diabetes intolerance.

In fact, a Mediterranean diet is far better than a low-fat diet when it comes to weight loss. Additionally, the diet has been linked to a reduction in the risk of chronic diseases like metabolic syndrome and type-2 diabetes.

Reducing the Risk of Cancer

Most ingredients used in a typical Mediterranean diet contain high levels of antioxidants, especially from colorful plant foods. Antioxidants are compounds that slow down or stop oxidative damage and reduce inflammation throughout the body. Hence, a Mediterranean diet is associated with a reduced risk of neurodegenerative diseases and cancer.

According to studies, it has been found that a Mediterranean diet provides a protective effect against different types of cancers. A particular research showed that a Mediterranean diet is particularly effective against certain types of cancers like gastric, colorectal, and breast cancers. Researchers have also concluded that a Mediterranean diet that contains whole grains, vegetables, and fruits are the best bet against cancer.

Improves Mood and Good for Your Memory

For the same reasons why, a Mediterranean diet is great for preventing cancer (i.e., it has anti-inflammatory and antioxidant properties), this diet is also great for improving brain health. Research has shown that a Mediterranean diet significantly reduces and/or delays the risk of depression and Alzheimer's disease. A Mediterranean diet consists of vegetables and fruits like melons, apricots, tomatoes, sweet potatoes, kale, spinach, and carrots that have higher carotenoid antioxidants; this has been linked to improving optimized and mood.

Improves Your Gut Health

A Mediterranean diet consists of vegetables, fruits, and whole grains; this means that this diet is full of antioxidants, minerals, vitamins, and fiber. All these nutrients benefit and improve gut health by feeding the beneficial probiotic bacteria that reside there and reduces inflammation as well. In a study done of primates that fed a plant-heavy Mediterranean diet, the animals had a higher population of good gut bacteria, than those that were given a meat-based Western diet. The health of your gut is closely related to your mental health, which is another reason why a Mediterranean diet improves mood.

BREAKFAST RECIPES

1. Smoked Salmon and Poached Eggs on Toast

Preparation Time: 10 minutes

Cooking Time: 4 minutes

Servings: 4

INGREDIENTS:

- 2 oz avocado smashed
- 2 slices of bread toasted
- Pinch of kosher salt and cracked black pepper
- 1/4 tsp freshly squeezed lemon juice
- 2 eggs see notes, poached
- 3.5 oz smoked salmon
- 1 TBSP. thinly sliced scallions
- Splash of Kikkoman soy sauce optional
- Microgreens are optional

DIRECTIONS:

1. Take a small bowl and then smash the avocado into it. Then, add the lemon juice and also a pinch of salt into the mixture. Then, mix it well and set aside.

2. After that, poach the eggs and toast the bread for some time. Once the bread is toasted, you will have to spread the avocado on both slices and after that, add the smoked salmon to each slice.

3. Thereafter, carefully transfer the poached eggs to the respective toasts. Add a splash of Kikkoman soy sauce and some cracked pepper; then, just garnish with scallions and microgreens.

NUTRITION: Calories: 459 Protein: 31 g Fat: 22 g Carbs: 33 g

2. <u>Honey Almond Ricotta Spread with Peaches</u>

Preparation Time: 5 minutes

Cooking Time: 8 minutes

Servings: 4

INGREDIENTS:

- 1/2 cup Fisher Sliced Almonds
- 1 cup whole milk ricotta
- 1/4 teaspoon almond extract
- zest from an orange, optional
- 1 teaspoon honey
- hearty whole-grain toast
- English muffin or bagel
- extra Fisher sliced almonds
- sliced peaches

- extra honey for drizzling

DIRECTIONS:

1. Cut peaches into a proper shape and then brush them with olive oil. After that, set it aside. Take a bowl; combine the ingredients for the filling. Set aside.
2. Then just pre-heat grill to medium. Place peaches cut side down onto the greased grill. Close lid cover and then just grill until the peaches have softened, approximately 6-10 minutes, depending on the size of the peaches.
3. Then you will have to place peach halves onto a serving plate. Put a spoon of about 1 tablespoon of ricotta mixture into the cavity (you are also allowed to use a small scooper).
4. Sprinkle it with slivered almonds, crushed amaretti cookies, and honey. Decorate with the mint leaves.

NUTRITION: Calories: 187 Protein: 7 g Fat: 9 g Carbs: 18 g

3. Mediterranean Eggs Cups

Preparation Time: 10 minutes

Cooking Time: 20 minutes

Servings: 8

INGREDIENTS:

- 1 cup spinach, finely diced
- 1/2 yellow onion, finely diced
- 1/2 cup sliced sun-dried tomatoes

- 4 large basil leaves, finely diced
- Pepper and salt to taste
- 1/3 cup feta cheese crumbles
- 8 large eggs
- 1/4 cup milk (any kind)

DIRECTIONS:

1. Warm the oven to 375°F. Then, roll the dough sheet into a 12x8-inch rectangle. Then, cut in half lengthwise.

2. After that, you will have to cut each half crosswise into 4 pieces, forming 8 (4x3-inch) pieces dough. Then, press each into the bottom and up sides of the ungreased muffin cup.

3. Trim dough to keep the dough from touching, if essential. Set aside. Then, you will have to combine the eggs, salt, pepper in the bowl and beat it with a whisk until well mixed. Set aside.

4. Melt the butter in 12-inch skillet over medium heat until sizzling; add bell peppers. You will have to cook it, stirring occasionally, 2-3 minutes or until crisply tender.

5. After that, add spinach leaves; continue cooking until spinach is wilted. Then just add egg mixture and prosciutto.

6. Divide the mixture evenly among prepared muffin cups. Finally, bake it for 14-17 minutes or until the crust is golden brown.

NUTRITION: Calories: 240 Protein: 9 g Fat: 16 g Carbs: 13 g

4. Low-Carb Baked Eggs with Avocado and Feta

Preparation Time: 10 minutes

Cooking Time: 15 minutes

Servings: 2

INGREDIENTS:

- 1 avocado
- 4 eggs
- 2-3 tbsp. crumbled feta cheese
- Nonstick cooking spray
- Pepper and salt to taste

DIRECTIONS:

1. First, you will have to preheat the oven to 400 degrees F. After that, when the oven is on the proper temperature, you will have to put the gratin dishes right on the baking sheet.
2. Then, leave the dishes to heat in the oven for almost 10 minutes After that process, you need to break the eggs into individual ramekins.
3. Then, let the avocado and eggs come to room temperature for at least 10 minutes. Then, peel the avocado properly and cut it each half into 6-8 slices.
4. You will have to remove the dishes from the oven and spray them with the non-stick spray. Then, you will have to arrange all

the sliced avocados in the dishes and tip two eggs into each dish. Sprinkle with feta, add pepper and salt to taste, serve.

NUTRITION: Calories: 280 Protein: 11 g Fat: 23 g Carbs: 10 g

5. Mediterranean Eggs White Breakfast Sandwich with Roasted Tomatoes

Preparation Time: 15 minutes

Cooking Time: 10 minutes

Servings: 2

INGREDIENTS:

- Salt and pepper to taste
- ¼ cup egg whites
- 1 teaspoon chopped fresh herbs like rosemary, basil, parsley,
- 1 whole-grain seeded ciabatta roll
- 1 teaspoon butter
- 1-2 slices Muenster cheese
- 1 tablespoon pesto
- About ½ cup roasted tomatoes
- 10 ounces grape tomatoes
- 1 tablespoon extra-virgin olive oil
- Black pepper and salt to taste

DIRECTIONS:

1. First, you will have to melt the butter over medium heat in the small nonstick skillet. Then, mix the egg whites with pepper and salt.

2. Then, sprinkle it with the fresh herbs. After that cook it for almost 3-4 minutes or until the eggs are done, then flip it carefully.

3. Meanwhile, toast ciabatta bread in the toaster. Place the egg on the bottom half of the sandwich rolls, then top with cheese

4. Add roasted tomatoes and the top half of roll. To make a roasted tomato, preheat the oven to 400 degrees. Then, slice the tomatoes in half lengthwise.

5. Place on the baking sheet and drizzle with olive oil. Season it with pepper and salt and then roast in the oven for about 20 minutes. Skins will appear wrinkled when done.

NUTRITION: Calories: 458 Protein: 21 g Fat: 24 g Carbs: 51 g

6. Greek Yogurt Pancakes

Preparation Time: 10 minutes

Cooking Time: 5 minutes

Servings: 2

INGREDIENTS:

- 1 cup all-purpose flour
- 1 cup whole-wheat flour
- 1/4 teaspoon salt
- 4 teaspoons baking powder

- 1 tablespoon sugar
- 1 1/2 cups unsweetened almond milk
- 2 teaspoons vanilla extract
- 2 large eggs
- 1/2 cup plain 2% Greek yogurt
- Fruit, for serving
- Maple syrup, for serving

DIRECTIONS:

1. First, you will have to pour the curds into the bowl and mix them well until creamy. After that, you will have to add egg whites and mix them well until combined.
2. Then take a separate bowl, pour the wet mixture into the dry mixture. Stir to combine. The batter will be extremely thick.
3. Then, simply spoon the batter onto the sprayed pan heated too medium-high. The batter must make 4 large pancakes.
4. Then, you will have to flip the pancakes once when they start to bubble a bit on the surface. Cook until golden brown on both sides.

NUTRITION: Calories: 166 Protein: 14 g Fat: 5 g Carbs: 52g

7. Mediterranean Feta and Quinoa Egg Muffins

Preparation Time: 15 minutes

Cooking Time: 15 minutes

Servings: 12

INGREDIENTS:

- 2 cups baby spinach finely chopped
- 1 cup chopped or sliced cherry tomatoes
- 1/2 cup finely chopped onion
- 1 tablespoon chopped fresh oregano
- 1 cup crumbled feta cheese
- 1/2 cup chopped {pitted} kalamata olives
- 2 teaspoons high oleic sunflower oil
- 1 cup cooked quinoa
- 8 eggs
- 1/4 teaspoon salt

DIRECTIONS:

1. Pre-heat oven to 350 degrees Fahrenheit, and then prepare 12 silicone muffin holders on the baking sheet, or just grease a 12-cup muffin tin with oil and set aside.
2. Finely chop the vegetables and then heat the skillet to medium. After that, add the vegetable oil and onions and sauté for 2 minutes.
3. Then, add tomatoes and sauté for another minute, then add spinach and sauté until wilted, about 1 minute.
4. Place the beaten egg into a bowl and then add lots of vegetables like feta cheese, quinoa, veggie mixture as well as salt, and then stir well until everything is properly combined.

5. Pour the ready mixture into greased muffin tins or silicone cups, dividing the mixture equally. Then, bake it in an oven for 30 minutes or so.

NUTRITION: Calories: 113 Protein: 6 g Fat: 7 g Carbs: 5 g

8. Mediterranean Eggs

Preparation Time: 15 minutes

Cooking Time: 20 minutes

Servings: 2

INGREDIENTS:

- 5 tbsp. of divided olive oil
- 2 diced medium-sized Spanish onions
- 2 diced red bell peppers
- 2 minced cloves garlic
- 1 teaspoon cumin seeds
- 4 diced large ripe tomatoes
- 1 tablespoon of honey
- Salt
- Freshly ground black pepper
- 1/3 cup crumbled feta
- 4 eggs
- 1 teaspoon zaatar spice
- Grilled pita during serving

DIRECTIONS:

1. Add 3 tablespoons of olive oil into a pan and heat it over medium heat. Along with the oil, sauté the cumin seeds, onions, garlic, and red pepper for a few minutes.

2. After that, add the diced tomatoes and salt and pepper to taste and cook them for about 10 minutes till they come together and form a light sauce.

3. With that, half the preparation is already done. Now you just have to break the eggs directly into the sauce and poach them.

4. However, you must keep in mind to cook the egg whites but keep the yolks still runny. This takes about 8 to 10 minutes.

5. While plating adds some feta and olive oil with zaatar spice to further enhance the flavors. Once done, serve with grilled pita.

NUTRITION: Calories: 304 Protein: 12 g Fat: 16 g Carbs: 28 g

9. Pastry-Less Spanakopita

Preparation Time: 5 minutes

Cooking Time: 20 minutes

Servings: 4

INGREDIENTS:

- 1/8 teaspoons black pepper, add as per taste
- 1/3 cup of Extra virgin olive oil
- 4 lightly beaten eggs
- 7 cups of Lettuce, preferably a spring mix (mesclun)
- 1/2 cup of crumbled Feta cheese

- 1/8 teaspoon of Sea salt, add to taste
- 1 finely chopped medium Yellow onion

DIRECTIONS:

1. Warm the oven to 180C and grease the flan dish. Once done, pour the extra virgin olive oil into a large saucepan and heat it over medium heat with the onions, until they are translucent.
2. Add greens and keep stirring until all the ingredients are wilted. Season it with salt and pepper and transfer the greens to the prepared dish and sprinkle on some feta cheese.
3. Pour the eggs and bake it for 20 minutes till it is cooked through and slightly brown.

NUTRITION: Calories: 325 Protein: 11.2 g Fat: 27.9 g Carbs: 7.3 g

10. Date and Walnut Overnight Oats

Preparation Time: 5 minutes

Cooking Time: 20 minutes

Servings: 2

INGREDIENTS:

- ¼ Cup Greek Yogurt, Plain
- 1/3 cup of yogurt
- 2/3 cup of oats
- 1 cup of milk
- 2 tsp date syrup or you can also use maple syrup or honey
- 1 mashed banana

- ¼ tsp cinnamon
- ¼ cup walnuts
- pinch of salt (approx.1/8 tsp)

DIRECTIONS:

1. Firstly, get a mason jar or a small bowl and add all the ingredients. After that stir and mix all the ingredients well. Cover it securely, and cool it in a refrigerator overnight.
2. After that, take it out the next morning, add more liquid or cinnamon if required, and serve cold. (However, you can also microwave it for people with a warmer palate.)

NUTRITION: Calories: 350 Protein: 14 g Fat: 12 g Carbs: 49 g

APPETIZER AND SNACK

RECIPES

---

11. Tomato Cream Cheese Spread

Preparation time: 15 minutes

Cooking Time: 0 Minutes

Servings: 6

INGREDIENTS:

- 12 ounces cream cheese, soft
- 1 big tomato, cubed
- ¼ cup homemade mayonnaise
- 2 garlic cloves, minced
- 2 tablespoons red onion, chopped
- 2 tablespoons lime juice
- Salt and black pepper to the taste

DIRECTIONS:

1. In your blender, mix the cream cheese with the tomato and the rest of the ingredients, pulse well, divide into small cups and serve cold.

NUTRITION: Calories 204 Fat 6.7g Carbs 7.3g Protein 4.5g

12. Italian Fries

Preparation time: 15 minutes

Cooking Time: 40 Minutes

Servings: 4

INGREDIENTS:

- 1/3 cup baby red potatoes
- 1 tablespoon Italian seasoning
- 3 tablespoons canola oil
- 1 teaspoon turmeric
- ½ teaspoon of sea salt
- ½ teaspoon dried rosemary
- 1 tablespoon dried dill

DIRECTIONS:

1. Cut the red potatoes into the wedges and transfer in the big bowl. After this, sprinkle the vegetables with Italian seasoning, canola oil, turmeric, sea salt, dried rosemary, and dried dill.
2. Shake the potato wedges carefully. Line the baking tray with baking paper. Place the potatoes wedges in the tray. Flatten it well to make one layer. Preheat the oven to 375F.
3. Place the tray with potatoes in the oven and bake for 40 minutes. Stir the potatoes with the help of the spatula from time to time. The potato fries are cooked when they have crunchy edges.

NUTRITION: Calories 122 Fat 11.6g Carbs 4.5g Protein 0.6g

13. Tempeh Snack

Preparation time: 15 minutes

Cooking Time: 8 Minutes

Servings: 6

INGREDIENTS:

- 11 oz soy tempeh
- 1 teaspoon olive oil
- ½ teaspoon ground black pepper
- ¼ teaspoon garlic powder

DIRECTIONS:

1. Cut soy tempeh into the sticks. Sprinkle every tempeh stick with ground black pepper, garlic powder, and olive oil. Preheat the grill to 375F.
2. Place the tempeh sticks in the grill and cook them for 4 minutes from each side. The time of cooking depends on the tempeh sticks size. The cooked tempeh sticks will have a light brown color.

NUTRITION: Calories 88 Fat 2.5g Carbs 10.2g Protein 6.5g

14. Avocado Dip

Preparation time: 15 minutes

Cooking Time: 0 Minutes

Servings: 8

INGREDIENTS:

- ½ cup heavy cream
- 1 green chili pepper, chopped
- Salt and pepper to the taste
- 4 avocados, pitted, peeled and chopped
- 1 cup cilantro, chopped
- ¼ cup lime juice

DIRECTIONS:

1. In a blender, combine the cream with the avocados and the rest of the ingredients and pulse well. Divide the mix into bowls and serve cold as a party dip.

NUTRITION: Calories 200 Fat 14.5g Carbs 8.1g Protein 7.6g

15. Feta and Roasted Red Pepper Bruschetta

Preparation time: 15 minutes

Cooking Time: 15 Minutes

Servings: 24

INGREDIENTS:

- 6 Kalamata olives, pitted, chopped
- 2 tablespoons green onion, minced

- 1/4 cup Parmesan cheese, grated, divided
- 1/4 cup extra-virgin olive oil brushing, or as needed
- 1/4 cup cherry tomatoes, thinly sliced
- 1 teaspoon lemon juice
- 1 tablespoon extra-virgin olive oil
- 1 tablespoon basil pesto
- 1 red bell pepper, halved, seeded
- 1 piece (12 inch) whole-wheat baguette, cut into 1/2-inch-thick slices
- 1 package (4 ounce) feta cheese with basil and sun-dried tomatoes, crumbled
- 1 clove garlic, minced

DIRECTIONS:

1. Preheat the oven broiler. Place the oven rack 6 inches from the source of heat. Brush both sides of the baguette slices, with the 1/4 cup olive oil.
2. Arrange the bread slices on a baking sheet; toast for about 1 minute each side, carefully watching to avoid burning. Remove the toasted slices, transferring into another baking sheet.
3. With the cut sides down, place the red peppers in a baking sheet; broil for about 8 to 10 minutes or until the skin is charred and blistered.
4. Transfer the roasted peppers into a bowl; cover with plastic wrap. Let cool, remove the charred skin. Discard skin and chop the roasted peppers.

5. In a bowl, mix the roasted red peppers, cherry tomatoes, feta cheese, green onion, olives, pesto, 1 tablespoon olive oil, garlic, and lemon juice.

6. Top each bread with 1 tablespoon of the roasted pepper mix, sprinkle lightly with the Parmesan cheese.

7. Return the baking sheet with the topped bruschetta; broil for about 1-2 minutes or until the topping is lightly browned.

NUTRITION: Cal 73 Fat 4.8 g Carbs 5.3 g Protein 2.1 g

16. Meat-Filled Phyllo (Samboosek)

Preparation time: 15 minutes

Cooking Time: 10 Minutes

Servings: 1 Phyllo Pie

INGREDIENTS:

- 1 lb. ground beef or lamb
- 1 medium yellow onion, finely chopped
- 1 tbsp seven spices
- 1 tsp. salt
- 1 pkg. frozen phyllo dough (12 sheets)
- 2/3 cup butter, melted

DIRECTIONS:

1. In a medium skillet over medium heat, brown beef for 3 minutes, breaking up chunks with a wooden spoon.

2. Add yellow onion, seven spices, and salt, and cook for 5 to 7 minutes or until beef is browned and onions are translucent. Set aside, and let cool.

3. Place first sheet of phyllo on your work surface, brush with melted butter, lay second sheet of phyllo on top, and brush with melted butter. Cut sheets into 3-inch-wide strips.

4. Spoon 2 tablespoons meat filling at end of each strip, and fold end strip to cover meat and form a triangle.

5. Fold pointed end up and over to the opposite end, and you should see a triangle forming. Continue to fold up and then over until you come to the end of strip.

6. Place phyllo pies on a baking sheet, seal side down, and brush tops with butter. Repeat with remaining phyllo and filling. Bake for 10 minutes or until golden brown.

7. Remove from the oven and set aside for 5 minutes before serving warm or at room temperature.

NUTRITION: Calories: 299 Carbs: 53g Fat: 6g Protein: 7g

17. Tasty Black Bean Dip

Preparation time: 15 minutes

Cooking Time: 18 Minutes

Servings: 6

INGREDIENTS:

- 2 cups dry black beans, soaked overnight and drained
- 1 1/2 cups cheese, shredded

- 1 tsp dried oregano
- 1 1/2 tsp chili powder
- 2 cups tomatoes, chopped
- 2 tbsp olive oil
- 1 1/2 tbsp garlic, minced
- 1 medium onion, sliced
- 4 cups vegetable stock
- Pepper
- Salt

DIRECTIONS:

1. Add all ingredients except cheese into the instant pot. Seal pot with lid and cook on high for 18 minutes. Once done, allow to release pressure naturally. Remove lid. Drain excess water.
2. Add cheese and stir until cheese is melted. Blend bean mixture using an immersion blender until smooth. Serve and enjoy.

NUTRITION: Calories 402 Fat 15.3 g Carbohydrates 46.6 g Protein 22.2 g

18. Zucchini Cakes

Preparation time: 15 minutes

Cooking Time: 10 Minutes

Servings: 4

INGREDIENTS:

- 1 zucchini, grated

- ¼ carrot, grated
- ¼ onion, minced
- 1 teaspoon minced garlic
- 3 tablespoons coconut flour
- 1 teaspoon Italian seasonings
- 1 egg, beaten
- 1 teaspoon coconut oil

DIRECTIONS:

1. In the mixing bowl combine together grated zucchini, carrot, minced onion, and garlic. Add coconut flour, Italian seasoning, and egg. Stir the mass until homogenous.
2. Heat up coconut oil in the skillet. Place the small zucchini fritters in the hot oil. Make them with the help of the spoon. Roast the zucchini fritters for 4 minutes from each side.

NUTRITION: Calories 65 Fat 3.3g Carbs 6.3g Protein 3.3g

19. Parsley Nachos

Preparation time: 15 minutes

Cooking Time: 0 Minutes

Servings: 3

INGREDIENTS:

- 3 oz tortilla chips
- ¼ cup Greek yogurt
- 1 tablespoon fresh parsley, chopped

- ¼ teaspoon minced garlic
- 2 kalamata olives, chopped
- 1 teaspoon paprika
- ¼ teaspoon ground thyme

DIRECTIONS:

1. In the mixing bowl mix up together Greek yogurt, parsley, minced garlic, olives, paprika, and thyme. Then add tortilla chips and mix up gently. The snack should be served immediately.

NUTRITION: Calories 81 Fat 1.6g Carbs 14.1g Protein 3.5g

20. Plum Wraps

Preparation time: 15 minutes

Cooking Time: 10 Minutes

Servings: 4

INGREDIENTS:

- 4 plums
- 4 prosciutto slices
- ¼ teaspoon olive oil

DIRECTIONS:

1. Preheat the oven to 375F. Wrap every plum in prosciutto slice and secure with a toothpick (if needed). Place the wrapped plums in the oven and bake for 10 minutes.

NUTRITION: Calories 62 Fat 2.2g Carbs 8g Protein 4.3g

21. Parmesan Chips

Preparation time: 15 minutes

Cooking Time: 20 Minutes

Servings: 4

INGREDIENTS:

- 1 zucchini
- 2 oz Parmesan, grated
- ½ teaspoon paprika
- 1 teaspoon olive oil

DIRECTIONS:

1. Trim zucchini and slice it into the chips with the help of the vegetable slices. Then mix up together Parmesan and paprika. Sprinkle the zucchini chips with olive oil.
2. After this, dip every zucchini slice in the cheese mixture. Place the zucchini chips in the lined baking tray and bake for 20 minutes at 375F.
3. Flip the zucchini sliced onto another side after 10 minutes of cooking. Chill the cooked chips well.

NUTRITION: Calories 64 Fat 4.3g Carbs 2.3g Protein 5.2g

22. Chicken Bites

Preparation time: 15 minutes

Cooking Time: 5 Minutes

Servings: 6

INGREDIENTS:

- ½ cup coconut flakes
- 8 oz chicken fillet
- ¼ cup Greek yogurt
- 1 teaspoon dried dill
- 1 teaspoon salt
- 1 teaspoon ground black pepper
- 1 tablespoon tomato sauce
- 1 teaspoon honey
- 4 tablespoons sunflower oil

DIRECTIONS:

1. Chop the chicken fillet on the small cubes (popcorn cubes). Sprinkle them with dried dill, salt, and ground black pepper.
2. Then add Greek yogurt and stir carefully. After this, pour sunflower oil in the skillet and heat it up.
3. Coat chicken cubes in the coconut flakes and roast in the hot oil for 3-4 minutes or until the popcorn cubes are golden brown.
4. Dry the popcorn chicken with the help of the paper towel. Make the sweet sauce: whisk together honey and tomato sauce. Serve the popcorn chicken hot or warm with sweet sauce.

NUTRITION: Calories 107 Fat 5.2g Carbs 2.8g Protein 12.1g

23. Chicken Kale Wraps

Preparation time: 15 minutes

Cooking Time: 10 Minutes

Servings: 4

INGREDIENTS:

- 4 kale leaves
- 4 oz chicken fillet
- ½ apple
- 1 tablespoon butter
- ¼ teaspoon chili pepper
- ¾ teaspoon salt
- 1 tablespoon lemon juice
- ¾ teaspoon dried thyme

DIRECTIONS:

1. Chop the chicken fillet into the small cubes. Then mix up together chicken with chili pepper and salt. Heat up butter in the skillet. Add chicken cubes. Roast them for 4 minutes.
2. Meanwhile, chop the apple into small cubes and add it in the chicken. Mix up well. Sprinkle the ingredients with lemon juice and dried thyme.
3. Cook them for 5 minutes over the medium-high heat. Fill the kale leaves with the hot chicken mixture and wrap.

NUTRITION: Calories 106 Fat 5.1 Carbs 6.3 Protein 9

24. Savory Pita Chips

Preparation time: 15 minutes

Cooking Time: 10 Minutes

Servings: 1 Cup

INGREDIENTS:

- 3 pitas
- 1/4 cup extra-virgin olive oil
- 1/4 cup zaatar

DIRECTIONS:

1. Preheat the oven to 450°F. Cut pitas into 2-inch pieces, and place in a large bowl. Drizzle pitas with extra-virgin olive oil, sprinkle with zaatar, and toss to coat.
2. Spread out pitas on a baking sheet, and bake for 8 to 10 minutes or until lightly browned and crunchy.
3. Let pita chips cool before removing from the baking sheet. Store in an airtight container for up to 1 month.

NUTRITION: Calories: 108 Carbs: 18g Fat: 2g Protein: 5g

25. Artichoke Skewers

Preparation time: 15 minutes

Cooking Time: 0 Minutes

Servings: 4

INGREDIENTS:

- 4 prosciutto slices
- 4 artichoke hearts, canned
- 4 kalamata olives
- 4 cherry tomatoes
- ¼ teaspoon cayenne pepper
- ¼ teaspoon sunflower oil

DIRECTIONS:

1. Skewer prosciutto slices, artichoke hearts, kalamata olives, and cherry tomatoes on the wooden skewers. Sprinkle antipasto skewers with sunflower oil and cayenne pepper.

NUTRITION: Calories 152 Fat 3.7g Carbs 23.2g Protein 11.1g

26. Kidney Bean Spread

Preparation time: 15 minutes

Cooking Time: 18 Minutes

Servings: 4

INGREDIENTS:

- 1 lb. dry kidney beans, soaked overnight and drained
- 1 tsp garlic, minced
- 2 tbsp olive oil
- 1 tbsp fresh lemon juice
- 1 tbsp paprika
- 4 cups vegetable stock

- 1/2 cup onion, chopped
- Pepper
- Salt

DIRECTIONS:

1. Add beans and stock into the instant pot. Seal pot with lid and cook on high for 18 minutes. Once done, allow to release pressure naturally. Remove lid.
2. Drain beans well and reserve 1/2 cup stock. Transfer beans, reserve stock, and remaining ingredients into the food processor and process until smooth. Serve and enjoy.

NUTRITION: Calories 461 Fat 8.6 g Carbohydrates 73 g Protein 26.4 g

27. Mediterranean Polenta Cups Recipe

Preparation time: 15 minutes

Cooking Time: 5 Minutes

Servings: 24

INGREDIENTS:

- 1 cup yellow cornmeal
- 1 garlic clove, minced
- 1/2 teaspoon fresh thyme, minced or 1/4 teaspoon dried thyme
- 1/2 teaspoon salt
- 1/4 cup feta cheese, crumbled
- 1/4 teaspoon pepper

- 2 tablespoons fresh basil, chopped
- 4 cups water
- 4 plum tomatoes, finely chopped

DIRECTIONS:

1. In a heavy, large saucepan, bring the water and the salt to a boil; reduce the heat to a gentle boil.

2. Slowly whisk in the cornmeal; cook, stirring with a wooden spoon for about 15 to 20 minutes, or until the polenta is thick and pulls away cleanly from the sides of the pan.

3. Remove from the heat; stir in the pepper and the thyme. Grease miniature muffin cups with cooking spray. Spoon a heaping tablespoon of the polenta mixture into each muffin cups.

4. With the back of a spoon, make an indentation in the center of each; cover and chill until the mixture is set.

5. Meanwhile, combine the feta cheese, tomatoes, garlic, and basil in a small-sized bowl. Unmold the chilled polenta cups; place them on an ungreased baking sheet.

6. Tops each indentation with 1 heaping tablespoon of the feta mixture. Broil the cups 4 inches from the heat source for about 5 to 7 minutes, or until heated through.

NUTRITION: Calories: 70 Carbs: 15g Fat: 0g Protein: 2g

28. Tomato Triangles

Preparation time: 15 minutes

Cooking Time: 0 Minutes

Servings: 6

INGREDIENTS:

- 6 corn tortillas
- 1 tablespoon cream cheese
- 1 tablespoon ricotta cheese
- ½ teaspoon minced garlic
- 1 tablespoon fresh dill, chopped
- 2 tomatoes, sliced

DIRECTIONS:

1. Cut every tortilla into 2 triangles. Then mix up together cream cheese, ricotta cheese, minced garlic, and dill.
2. Spread 6 triangles with cream cheese mixture. Then place sliced tomato on them and cover with remaining tortilla triangles.

NUTRITION: Calories 71 Fat 1.6g Carbs 12.8g Protein 2.3g

29. Chili Mango and Watermelon Salsa

Preparation time: 15 minutes

Cooking Time: 0 Minutes

Servings: 12

INGREDIENTS:

- 1 red tomato, chopped
- Salt and black pepper to the taste
- 1 cup watermelon, seedless, peeled and cubed

- 1 red onion, chopped
- 2 mangos, peeled and chopped
- 2 chili peppers, chopped
- ¼ cup cilantro, chopped
- 3 tablespoons lime juice
- Pita chips for serving

DIRECTIONS:

1. In a bowl, mix the tomato with the watermelon, the onion and the rest of the ingredients except the pita chips and toss well. Divide the mix into small cups and serve with pita chips on the side.

NUTRITION: Calories 62 Fat 4.7g Carbs 3.9g Protein 2.3g

30. Tomato Olive Salsa

Preparation time: 15 minutes

Cooking Time: 5 Minutes

Servings: 4

INGREDIENTS:

- 2 cups olives, pitted and chopped
- 1/4 cup fresh parsley, chopped
- 1/4 cup fresh basil, chopped
- 2 tbsp green onion, chopped
- 1 cup grape tomatoes, halved

- 1 tbsp olive oil
- 1 tbsp vinegar
- Pepper
- Salt

DIRECTIONS:

1. Add all ingredients into the inner pot of instant pot and stir well. Seal pot with lid and cook on high for 5 minutes.
2. Once done, allow to release pressure naturally for 5 minutes then release remaining using quick release. Remove lid. Stir well and serve.

NUTRITION: Calories 119 Fat 10.8 g Carbohydrates 6.5 g Protein 1.2 g

SOUP RECIPES

31. Cheesy Chicken Soup

Preparation Time: 10 minutes

Cooking Time: 15 minutes

Servings: 4

INGREDIENTS:

- 12 oz chicken thighs, boneless
- 1 cup heavy cream
- 2 cups cheddar cheese, shredded
- 3 cups chicken stock
- 2 tbsp olive oil
- 1/2 cup celery, chopped
- 1/4 cup hot sauce
- 1 tsp garlic, minced
- 1/4 cup onion, chopped

DIRECTIONS:

1. Add all ingredients except cream and cheese into the instant pot and stir well. Seal pot with lid and cook on high pressure 15 for minutes.

2. Once done, allow to release pressure naturally. Remove lid. Shred the chicken using a fork. Add cream and cheese and stir until cheese is melted. Serve and enjoy.

NUTRITION: Calories 568 Fat 43.6 g Carbohydrates 3.6 g Protein 40.1 g

32. Creamy Cauliflower Soup

Preparation Time: 10 minutes

Cooking Time: 23 minutes

Servings: 4

INGREDIENTS:

- 1 lb. cauliflower florets, chopped
- 2 tbsp fresh chives, chopped
- 1 tsp curry powder
- 2 cups vegetable stock
- 14 oz coconut cream
- 1 onion, chopped
- 1 tbsp garlic, minced
- 1 tbsp olive oil
- Pepper
- Salt

DIRECTIONS:

1. Add oil into the inner pot of instant pot and set the pot on sauté mode. Add onion and garlic and sauté for 3 minutes. Add the rest of the ingredients and stir well.

2. Seal pot with lid and cook on high for 20 minutes. Once done, allow to release pressure naturally for 10 minutes then release remaining using quick release. Remove lid.

3. Blend soup using an immersion blender until smooth. Serve and enjoy.

NUTRITION: Calories 306 Fat 27.4 g Carbohydrates 15.6 g Protein 5.3 g

33. **Delicious Okra Chicken Stew**

Preparation Time: 10 minutes

Cooking Time: 20 minutes

Servings: 4

INGREDIENTS:

- 1 lb. chicken breasts, skinless, boneless, and cubed
- 1 lemon juice
- 1/4 cup fresh parsley, chopped
- 1 tbsp olive oil
- 12 oz can tomato, crushed
- 1 tsp allspice
- 14 oz okra, chopped
- 2 cups chicken stock

- 1 tsp garlic, minced
- 1 onion, chopped
- Pepper
- Salt

DIRECTIONS:

1. Add oil into the inner pot of instant pot and set the pot on sauté mode. Add chicken and onion and sauté until chicken is lightly brown about 5 minutes.
2. Add remaining ingredients except for the parsley and stir well. Seal pot with lid and cook on high pressure 15 for minutes.
3. Once done, allow to release pressure naturally for 10 minutes then release remaining using quick release. Remove lid. Stir well and serve.

NUTRITION: Calories 326 Fat 12.6 g Carbohydrates 15.8 g Protein 36.4 g

34. Healthy Vegetable Soup

Preparation Time: 10 minutes

Cooking Time: 15 minutes

Servings: 4

INGREDIENTS:

1. 1 cup can tomato, chopped
2. 1 small zucchini, diced
3. 3 oz kale, sliced

4. 1 tbsp garlic, chopped

5. 5 button mushrooms, sliced

6. 2 carrots, peeled and sliced

7. 2 celery sticks, sliced

8. 1/2 red chili, sliced

9. 1 onion, diced

10. 1 tbsp olive oil

11. 1 bay leaf

12. 4 cups vegetable stock

13. 1/4 tsp salt

DIRECTIONS:

1. Add oil into the inner pot of instant pot and set the pot on sauté mode. Add carrots, celery, onion, and salt and cook for 2-3 minutes.

2. Add mushrooms and chili and cook for 2 minutes. Add remaining ingredients and stir everything well. Seal pot with lid and cook on high for 10 minutes.

3. Once done, allow to release pressure naturally for 10 minutes then release remaining using quick release. Remove lid. Stir well and serve.

NUTRITION: Calories 100 Fat 3.8 g Carbohydrates 15.1 g Protein 3.5 g

35. Spinach Chicken Stew

Preparation Time: 10 minutes

Cooking Time: 25 minutes

Servings: 4

INGREDIENTS:

- 2 cups spinach, chopped
- 1 lb., chicken breasts, skinless, boneless, and cut into chunks
- 1/2 cup can tomato, crushed
- 1 cup chicken stock
- 1 onion, chopped
- 1 tbsp olive oil
- Pepper
- Salt

DIRECTIONS:

1. Add oil into the inner pot of instant pot and set the pot on sauté mode. Add chicken and onion and sauté for 5 minutes. Add remaining ingredients and stir well.
2. Seal pot with lid and cook on low for 20 minutes. Once done, allow to release pressure naturally for 10 minutes then release remaining using quick release. Remove lid. Stir well and serve.

NUTRITION: Calories 266 Fat 12.2 g Carbohydrates 4.2 g Protein 33.9 g

36. Spinach Lentil Soup

Preparation Time: 10 minutes

Cooking Time: 30 minutes

Servings: 4

INGREDIENTS:

- 4 cups spinach
- 2 cups green lentils
- 4 cups vegetable stock
- 1 tsp Italian seasoning
- 14 oz can tomato, chopped
- 2 tsp thyme, chopped
- 1 tsp garlic, minced
- 1 carrot, chopped
- 1 onion, chopped
- 1 celery stalks, chopped
- Pepper
- Salt

DIRECTIONS:

1. Add all ingredients except spinach into the inner pot of instant pot and stir well. Seal pot with lid and cook on high for 25 minutes.
2. Once done, allow to release pressure naturally for 10 minutes then release remaining using quick release. Remove lid.
3. Add spinach and stir well and cook on sauté mode for 5 minutes. Stir well and serve.

NUTRITION: Calories 398 Fat 1.7 g Carbohydrates 69.8 g Protein 27.5 g

37. Basil Broccoli Soup

Preparation Time: 10 minutes

Cooking Time: 15 minutes

Servings: 6

INGREDIENTS:

- 1 lb. broccoli florets
- 1 tbsp olive oil
- 1 tsp chili powder
- 1 tsp dried basil
- 6 cups vegetable stock
- 1 onion, chopped
- 2 leeks, chopped
- Pepper
- Salt

DIRECTIONS:

1. Add oil into the inner pot of instant pot and set the pot on sauté mode. Add onion and leek and sauté for 5 minutes.
2. Add the rest of the ingredients and stir well. Seal pot with lid and cook on high for 10 minutes.
3. Once done, allow to release pressure naturally for 10 minutes then release remaining using quick release. Remove lid.
4. Blend soup using an immersion blender until smooth. Serve and enjoy.

NUTRITION: Calories 79 Fat 2.9 g Carbohydrates 12.1 g Protein 3.2 g

38. Basil Zucchini Soup

Preparation Time: 10 minutes

Cooking Time: 15 minutes

Servings: 4

INGREDIENTS:

- 1 zucchini, chopped
- 2 tbsp fresh basil, chopped
- 30 oz vegetable stock
- 1 tbsp garlic, minced
- 2 cups tomatoes, chopped
- 1 1/2 cup corn
- 1 onion, chopped
- 1 celery stalk, chopped
- 1 tbsp olive oil
- Pepper Salt

DIRECTIONS:

1. Add oil into the inner pot of instant pot and set the pot on sauté mode. Add onion and garlic and sauté for 5 minutes.
2. Add remaining ingredients except for basil and stir well. Seal pot with lid and cook on high for 10 minutes.

3. Once done, allow to release pressure naturally for 10 minutes then release remaining using quick release. Remove lid. Stir in basil and serve.

NUTRITION: Calories 139 Fat 4.8 g Carbohydrates 23 g Protein 5.2 g

39. Mushroom Carrot Soup

Preparation Time: 10 minutes

Cooking Time: 20 minutes

Servings: 4

INGREDIENTS:

- 16 oz mushrooms, sliced
- 1 carrot, chopped
- 4 cups vegetable stock
- 1 tsp dried thyme
- 1 tbsp garlic, minced
- 1 onion, chopped
- 1 celery stalk, chopped
- 1 tbsp olive oil
- Pepper Salt

DIRECTIONS:

1. Add oil into the inner pot of instant pot and set the pot on sauté mode. Add onion, garlic, celery, and carrot and sauté for 5 minutes.

2. Add mushrooms and sauté for 5 minutes. Add the rest of the ingredients and stir well. Seal pot with lid and cook on high for 10 minutes.

3. Once done, allow to release pressure naturally for 10 minutes then release remaining using quick release. Remove lid.

4. Blend soup using an immersion blender until smooth. Serve and enjoy.

NUTRITION: Calories 82 Fat 4 g Carbohydrates 9.7 g Protein 4.6 g

40. <u>Tomato Pepper Soup</u>

Preparation Time: 10 minutes

Cooking Time: 20 minutes

Servings: 4

INGREDIENTS:

- 1 lb. tomatoes, chopped
- 2 red bell peppers, chopped
- 1/2 tsp red pepper flakes
- 1/2 tbsp dried basil
- 1 tsp garlic powder
- 6 cups vegetable stock
- 2 celery stalks, chopped
- 3 tbsp tomato paste
- 1 onion, chopped
- 2 tbsp olive oil

- Pepper
- Salt

DIRECTIONS:

1. Add oil into the inner pot of instant pot and set the pot on sauté mode. Add onion, red pepper flakes, basil, and garlic powder and sauté for 5 minutes.
2. Add remaining ingredients and stir well. Seal pot with lid and cook on high for 15 minutes. Once done, allow to release pressure naturally for 10 minutes then release remaining using quick release. Remove lid.
3. Blend soup using an immersion blender until smooth. Serve and enjoy.

NUTRITION: Calories 134 Fat 7.7 g Carbohydrates 16 g Protein 3.2 g

MAIN RECIPES: MEAT

41. Cumin Lamb Mix

Preparation time: 15 minutes

Cooking Time: 10 Minutes

Servings: 2

INGREDIENTS:

- 2 lamb chops (3.5 oz each)
- 1 tablespoon olive oil
- 1 teaspoon ground cumin
- ½ teaspoon salt

DIRECTIONS:

1. Rub the lamb chops with ground cumin and salt. Then sprinkle them with olive oil. Let the meat marinate for 10 minutes. After this, preheat the skillet well.

2. Place the lamb chops in the skillet and roast them for 10 minutes. Flip the meat on another side from time to time to avoid burning.

NUTRITION: Calories 384 Fat 33.2g Carbs 0.5g Protein 19.2g

42. Beef & Potatoes

Preparation time: 15 minutes

Cooking Time: 20 Minutes

Servings: 6

INGREDIENTS:

- 1 1/2 lb. stew beef, sliced into cubes
- 2 teaspoons mixed dried herbs (thyme, sage)
- 4 potatoes, cubed
- 10 oz. mushrooms
- 1 ½ cups red wine

DIRECTIONS:

1. Set the Instant Pot to sauté. Add 1 tablespoon olive oil and cook the beef until brown on all sides. Add the rest of the ingredients.
2. Season with salt and pepper. Pour in 1 ½ cups water into the pot. Mix well. Cover the pot. Set it too manual. Cook at high pressure for 20 minutes. Release the pressure naturally.

NUTRITION: Calories 360 Fat 9.6g Carbohydrate 29.3g Protein 29.9g

43. Pork and Chestnuts Mix

Preparation time: 15 minutes

Cooking Time: 0 Minutes

Servings: 6

INGREDIENTS:

- 1 and ½ cups brown rice, already cooked
- 2 cups pork roast, already cooked and shredded
- 3 ounces water chestnuts, drained and sliced
- ½ cup sour cream
- A pinch of salt and white pepper

DIRECTIONS:

1. In a bowl, mix the rice with the roast and the other ingredients, toss and keep in the fridge for 2 hours before serving.

NUTRITION: Calories 294 Fat 17g Carbs 16g Protein 23.5g

44. Rosemary Pork Chops

Preparation time: 15 minutes

Cooking Time: 25 Minutes

Servings: 4

INGREDIENTS:

- 4 pork loin chops, boneless
- Salt and black pepper to the taste
- 4 garlic cloves, minced
- 1 tablespoon rosemary, chopped
- 1 tablespoon olive oil

DIRECTIONS:

1. In a roasting pan, combine the pork chops with the rest of the ingredients, toss, and bake at 425 degrees F for 10 minutes.
2. Reduce the heat to 350 degrees F and cook the chops for 25 minutes more. Divide the chops between plates and serve with a side salad.

NUTRITION: Calories 161 Fat 5g Carbs 1g Protein 25g

45. Tender Lamb

Preparation time: 45 minutes

Cooking Time: 40 Minutes

Servings: 6

INGREDIENTS:

- 3 lamb shanks
- Seasoning mixture (1 tablespoon oregano, 1/4 teaspoon ground cumin and 1 tablespoon smoked paprika)
- 3 cloves garlic, minced
- 2 cups red wine
- 4 cups beef stock

DIRECTIONS:

1. Coat the lamb shanks with the seasoning mixture. Sprinkle with salt and pepper. Cover with minced garlic. Marinate in half of the mixture for 30 minutes.

2. Set the Instant Pot to sauté. Pour in 2 tablespoons of olive oil. Brown the lamb on all sides. Remove and set aside. Add the rest of the ingredients.

3. Put the lamb back to the pot. Cover the pot and set it too manual. Cook at high pressure for 30 minutes. Release the pressure naturally. Set the Instant Pot to sauté to simmer and thicken the sauce.

NUTRITION: Calories 566 Fat 29.4g Carbohydrate 12g Protein 48.7g

46. **Worcestershire Pork Chops**

Preparation time: 15 minutes

Cooking Time: 15 Minutes

Servings: 3

INGREDIENTS:

- 2 tablespoons Worcestershire sauce
- 8 oz pork loin chops
- 1 tablespoon lemon juice
- 1 teaspoon olive oil

DIRECTIONS:

1. Mix up together Worcestershire sauce, lemon juice, and olive oil. Brush the pork loin chops with the sauce mixture from each side. Preheat the grill to 395F.

2. Place the pork chops in the grill and cook them for 5 minutes. Then flip the pork chops on another side and brush with remaining sauce mixture. Grill the meat for 7-8 minutes more.

NUTRITION: Calories 267 Fat 20.4g Carbs 2.1g Protein 17g

47. Greek Pork

Preparation time: 15 minutes

Cooking Time: 50 Minutes

Servings: 8

INGREDIENTS:

- 3 lb. pork roast, sliced into cubes
- 1/4 cup chicken broth
- 1/4 cup lemon juice
- 2 teaspoons dried oregano
- 2 teaspoons garlic powder

DIRECTIONS:

1. Put the pork in the Instant Pot. In a bowl, mix all the remaining ingredients. Pour the mixture over the pork. Toss to coat evenly. Secure the pot.
2. Choose manual mode. Cook at high pressure for 50 minutes. Release the pressure naturally.

NUTRITION: Calories 478 Fat 21.6g Carbohydrate 1.2g Protein 65.1g

48. **Pork with Green Beans & Potatoes**

Preparation time: 15 minutes

Cooking Time: 22 Minutes

Servings: 6

INGREDIENTS:

- 1 lb. lean pork, sliced into cubes
- 1 onion, chopped
- 2 carrots, sliced thinly
- 2 cups canned crushed tomatoes
- 2 potatoes, cubed

DIRECTIONS:

1. Set the Instant Pot to sauté. Add ½ cup of olive oil. Cook the pork for 5 minutes, stirring frequently. Add the rest of the ingredients. Mix well.
2. Seal the pot. Choose manual setting. Cook at high pressure for 17 minutes. Release the pressure naturally.

NUTRITION: Calories 428 Fat 24.4g Carbohydrate 27.6g Protein 26.7g

49. **Beef and Chili Mix**

Preparation time: 15 minutes

Cooking Time: 16 Minutes

Servings: 4

INGREDIENTS:

- 2 green chili peppers
- 8 oz beef flank steak
- 1 teaspoon salt
- 2 tablespoons olive oil
- 1 teaspoon apple cider vinegar

DIRECTIONS:

1. Pour olive oil in the skillet. Place the flank steak in the oil and roast it for 3 minutes from each side. Then sprinkle the meat with salt and apple cider vinegar.
2. Chop the chili peppers and add them in the skillet. Fry the beef for 10 minutes more. Stir it from time to time.

NUTRITION: Calories 166 Fat 10.5g Carbs 0.2g Protein17.2g

50. Greek Meatballs

Preparation time: 15 minutes

Cooking Time: 10 Minutes

Servings: 8-10

INGREDIENTS:

- 2 lb. ground lamb
- 1 onion, chopped
- 1/4 cup fresh parsley, chopped
- 1/2 cup almond flour

- 1 teaspoon dried oregano

DIRECTIONS:

1. In a large bowl, combine all the ingredients. Mix well and form into small meatballs. Put the balls on the steamer basket inside the Instant Pot.

2. Pour in 1 cup of broth to the bottom of the pot. Secure the pot. Choose manual. Cook at high pressure for 10 minutes. Release the pressure quickly. While waiting, mix the rest of the ingredients.

NUTRITION: Calories 214 Fat 7.9g Carbohydrate 5.5g Protein 28.7g

MAIN RECIPES: SEAFOOD

51. Salmon Baked in Foil

Preparation time: 5 minutes

Cooking time: 25 minutes

Servings: 4

INGREDIENTS:

- 2 cups cherry tomatoes
- 3 tablespoons extra-virgin olive oil
- 3 tablespoons lemon juice
- 3 tablespoons almond butter
- 1 teaspoon oregano
- ½ teaspoon salt
- 4 (5-ounce / 142-g) salmon fillets

DIRECTIONS:

1. Preheat the oven to 400°F (205°C). Cut the tomatoes in half and put them in a bowl. Add the olive oil, lemon juice, butter, oregano, and salt to the tomatoes and gently toss to combine.
2. Cut 4 pieces of foil, about 12-by-12 inches each. Place the salmon fillets in the middle of each piece of foil.

3. Divide the tomato mixture evenly over the 4 pieces of salmon. Bring the ends of the foil together and seal to form a closed pocket.

4. Place the 4 pockets on a baking sheet. Bake in the preheated oven for 25 minutes. Remove from the oven and serve on a plate.

NUTRITION: Calories: 410 Fat: 32.0g Protein: 30.0g Carbs: 4.0g

52. Instant Pot Poached Salmon

Preparation time: 10 minutes

Cooking time: 3 minutes

Servings: 4

INGREDIENTS:

- 1 lemon, sliced ¼ inch thick
- 4 (6-ounce / 170-g) skinless salmon fillets, 1½ inches thick
- ½ teaspoon salt
- ¼ teaspoon pepper
- ½ cup water

DIRECTIONS:

1. Layer the lemon slices in the bottom of the Instant Pot. Season the salmon with salt and pepper, then arrange the salmon (skin-side down) on top of the lemon slices. Pour in the water.

2. Secure the lid. Select the Manual mode and set the cooking time for 3 minutes at High Pressure. Once cooking is complete, do a quick pressure release. Carefully open the lid. Serve warm.

NUTRITION: Calories: 350 Fat: 23.0g Protein: 35.0g Carbs: 0g

53. Balsamic-Honey Glazed Salmon

Preparation time: 5 minutes

Cooking time: 8 minutes

Servings: 4

INGREDIENTS:

- ½ cup balsamic vinegar
- 1 tablespoon honey
- 4 (8-ounce / 227-g) salmon fillets
- Sea salt and freshly ground pepper, to taste
- 1 tablespoon olive oil

DIRECTIONS:

1. Heat a skillet over medium-high heat. Combine the vinegar and honey in a small bowl. Season the salmon fillets with the sea salt and freshly ground pepper; brush with the honey-balsamic glaze.
2. Add olive oil to the skillet, and sear the salmon fillets, cooking for 3 to 4 minutes on each side until lightly browned and medium rare in the center. Let sit for 5 minutes before serving.

NUTRITION: Calories: 454 Fat: 17.3g Protein: 65.3g Carbs: 9.7g

54. Seared Salmon with Lemon Cream Sauce

Preparation time: 10 minutes

Cooking time: 20 minutes

Servings: 4

INGREDIENTS:

- 4 (5-ounce / 142-g) salmon fillets
- Sea salt and freshly ground black pepper, to taste
- 1 tablespoon extra-virgin olive oil
- ½ cup low-sodium vegetable broth
- Juice and zest of 1 lemon
- 1 teaspoon chopped fresh thyme
- ½ cup fat-free sour cream
- 1 teaspoon honey
- 1 tablespoon chopped fresh chives

DIRECTIONS:

1. Preheat the oven to 400°F (205°C). Season the salmon lightly on both sides with salt and pepper. Place a large ovenproof skillet over medium-high heat and add the olive oil.

2. Sear the salmon fillets on both sides until golden, about 3 minutes per side. Transfer the salmon to a baking dish and bake in the preheated oven until just cooked through, about 10 minutes.

3. Meanwhile, whisk together the vegetable broth, lemon juice and zest, and thyme in a small saucepan over medium-high heat until the liquid reduces by about one-quarter, about 5 minutes.

4. Whisk in the sour cream and honey. Stir in the chives and serve the sauce over the salmon.

NUTRITION: Calories: 310 Fat: 18.0g Protein: 29.0g Carbs: 6.0g

55. Tuna and Zucchini Patties

Preparation time: 15 minutes

Cooking time: 12 minutes

Servings: 4

INGREDIENTS:

- 3 slices whole-wheat sandwich bread, toasted
- 2 (5-ounce / 142-g) cans tuna in olive oil, drained
- 1 cup shredded zucchini
- 1 large egg, lightly beaten
- ¼ cup diced red bell pepper
- 1 tablespoon dried oregano
- 1 teaspoon lemon zest
- ¼ teaspoon freshly ground black pepper
- ¼ teaspoon kosher or sea salt
- 1 tablespoon extra-virgin olive oil
- Salad greens or 4 whole-wheat rolls, for serving (optional)

DIRECTIONS:

1. Crumble the toast into bread crumbs with your fingers (or use a knife to cut into ¼-inch cubes) until you have 1 cup of loosely packed crumbs.

2. Pour the crumbs into a large bowl. Add the tuna, zucchini, beaten egg, bell pepper, oregano, lemon zest, black pepper, and salt. Mix well with a fork.

3. With your hands, form the mixture into four (½-cup-size) patties. Place them on a plate, and press each patty flat to about ¾-inch thick.

4. In a large skillet over medium-high heat, heat the oil until it's very hot, about 2 minutes. Add the patties to the hot oil, then reduce the heat down to medium.

5. Cook the patties for 5 minutes, flip with a spatula, and cook for an additional 5 minutes. Serve the patties on salad greens or whole-wheat rolls, if desired.

NUTRITION: Calories: 757 Fat: 72.0g Protein: 5.0g Carbs: 26.0g

56. Fennel Poached Cod with Tomatoes

Preparation time: 15 minutes

Cooking time: 20 minutes

Servings: 4

INGREDIENTS:

- 1 tablespoon olive oil
- 1 cup thinly sliced fennel
- ½ cup thinly sliced onion

- 1 tablespoon minced garlic
- 1 (15-ounce / 425-g) can diced tomatoes
- 2 cups chicken broth
- ½ cup white wine
- Juice and zest of 1 orange
- 1 pinch red pepper flakes
- 1 bay leaf
- 1 pound (454 g) cod

DIRECTIONS:

1. Heat the olive oil in a large skillet. Add the onion and fennel and cook for 6 minutes, stirring occasionally, or until translucent. Add the garlic and cook for 1 minute more.

2. Add the tomatoes, chicken broth, wine, orange juice and zest, red pepper flakes, and bay leaf, and simmer for 5 minutes to meld the flavors.

3. Carefully add the cod in a single layer, cover, and simmer for 6 to 7 minutes. Transfer fish to a serving dish, ladle the remaining sauce over the fish, and serve.

NUTRITION: Calories: 336 Fat: 12.5g Protein: 45.1g Carbs: 11.0g

57. Baked Fish with Pistachio Crust

Preparation time: 15 minutes

Cooking time: 15-20 minutes

Servings: 4

INGREDIENTS:

- ½ cup extra-virgin olive oil, divided
- 1 pound (454 g) flaky white fish (such as cod, haddock, or halibut), skin removed
- ½ cup shelled finely chopped pistachios
- ½ cup ground flaxseed
- Zest and juice of 1 lemon, divided
- 1 teaspoon ground cumin
- 1 teaspoon ground allspice
- ½ teaspoon salt
- ¼ teaspoon freshly ground black pepper

DIRECTIONS:

1. Preheat the oven to 400°F (205°C). Line a baking sheet with parchment paper or aluminum foil and drizzle 2 tablespoons of olive oil over the sheet, spreading to evenly coat the bottom.
2. Cut the fish into 4 equal pieces and place on the prepared baking sheet.
3. In a small bowl, combine the pistachios, flaxseed, lemon zest, cumin, allspice, salt, and pepper. Drizzle in ¼ cup of olive oil and stir well.
4. Divide the nut mixture evenly on top of the fish pieces. Drizzle the lemon juice and remaining 2 tablespoons of olive oil over the fish and bake until cooked through, 15 to 20 minutes, depending on the thickness of the fish. Cool for 5 minutes before serving.

NUTRITION: Calories: 509 Fat: 41.0g Protein: 26.0g Carbs: 9.0g

58. Dill Baked Sea Bass

Preparation time: 15 minutes

Cooking time: 10-15 minutes

Servings: 6

INGREDIENTS:

- ¼ cup olive oil
- 2 pounds (907 g) sea bass
- Sea salt and freshly ground pepper, to taste
- 1 garlic clove, minced
- ¼ cup dry white wine
- 3 teaspoons fresh dill
- 2 teaspoons fresh thyme

DIRECTIONS:

1. Preheat the oven to 425°F (220°C). Brush the bottom of a roasting pan with the olive oil. Place the fish in the pan and brush the fish with oil.
2. Season the fish with sea salt and freshly ground pepper. Combine the remaining ingredients and pour over the fish.
3. Bake in the preheated oven for 10 to 15 minutes, depending on the size of the fish. Serve hot.

NUTRITION: Calories: 224 Fat: 12.1g Protein: 28.1g Carbs: 0.9g

59. Sole Piccata with Capers

Preparation time: 15 minutes

Cooking time: 17 minutes

Servings: 4

INGREDIENTS:

- 1 teaspoon extra-virgin olive oil
- 4 (5-ounce / 142-g) sole fillets, patted dry
- 3 tablespoons almond butter
- 2 teaspoons minced garlic
- 2 tablespoons all-purpose flour
- 2 cups low-sodium chicken broth
- Juice and zest of ½ lemon
- 2 tablespoons capers

DIRECTIONS:

1. Place a large skillet over medium-high heat and add the olive oil. Sear the sole fillets until the fish flakes easily when tested with a fork, about 4 minutes on each side. Transfer the fish to a plate and set aside.

2. Return the skillet to the stove and add the butter. Sauté the garlic until translucent, about 3 minutes.

3. Whisk in the flour to make a thick paste and cook, stirring constantly, until the mixture is golden brown, about 2 minutes.

4. Whisk in the chicken broth, lemon juice and zest. Cook for about 4 minutes until the sauce is thickened. Stir in the capers and serve the sauce over the fish.

NUTRITION: Calories: 271 Fat: 13.0g Protein: 30.0g Carbs: 7.0g

60. Haddock with Cucumber Sauce

Preparation time: 15 minutes

Cooking time: 10 minutes

Servings: 4

INGREDIENTS:

- ¼ cup plain Greek yogurt
- ½ scallion, white and green parts, finely chopped
- ½ English cucumber, grated, liquid squeezed out
- 2 teaspoons chopped fresh mint
- 1 teaspoon honey
- Sea salt and freshly ground black pepper, to taste
- 4 (5-ounce / 142-g) haddock fillets, patted dry
- Nonstick cooking spray

DIRECTIONS:

1. In a small bowl, stir together the yogurt, cucumber, scallion, mint, honey, and a pinch of salt. Set aside. Season the fillets lightly with salt and pepper.

2. Place a large skillet over medium-high heat and spray lightly with cooking spray. Cook the haddock, turning once, until it is just cooked through, about 5 minutes per side.

3. Remove the fish from the heat and transfer to plates. Serve topped with the cucumber sauce.

NUTRITION: Calories: 164 Fat: 2.0g Protein: 27.0g Carbs: 4.0g

61. <u>**Crispy Herb Crusted Halibut**</u>

Preparation time: 15 minutes

Cooking time: 20 minutes

Servings: 4

INGREDIENTS:

- 4 (5-ounce / 142-g) halibut fillets, patted dry
- Extra-virgin olive oil, for brushing
- ½ cup coarsely ground unsalted pistachios
- 1 tablespoon chopped fresh parsley
- 1 teaspoon chopped fresh basil
- 1 teaspoon chopped fresh thyme
- Pinch sea salt
- Pinch freshly ground black pepper

DIRECTIONS:

1. Preheat the oven to 350°F (180°C). Line a baking sheet with parchment paper. Place the fillets on the baking sheet and brush them generously with olive oil.

2. In a small bowl, stir together the pistachios, parsley, basil, thyme, salt, and pepper. Spoon the nut mixture evenly on the fish, spreading it out so the tops of the fillets are covered.

3. Bake in the preheated oven until it flakes when pressed with a fork, about 20 minutes. Serve immediately.

NUTRITION: Calories: 262 Fat: 11.0g Protein: 32.0g Carbs: 4.0g

MAIN RECIPES

VEGETABLES

---

62. Easy Chili Pepper Zucchinis

Preparation time: 15 minutes

Cooking time: 10 minutes

Servings: 4

INGREDIENTS:

- 4 zucchinis, cut into cubes
- ½ teaspoon red pepper flakes
- ½ teaspoon cayenne
- 1 tablespoon chili powder
- ¼ cup vegetable stock
- Salt

DIRECTIONS:

1. Add all ingredients into the inner pot of instant pot and stir well. Seal pot with lid and cook on high for 10 minutes.
2. Once done, allow to release pressure naturally for 10 minutes then release remaining using quick release. Remove lid. Stir and serve.

NUTRITION: Calories: 38 Fat: 0.7 g Carbs: 8.8 g Protein: 2.7 g

63. Creamy Kale and Mushrooms

Preparation time: 15 minutes

Cooking time: 15 minutes

Servings: 3

INGREDIENTS:

- 3 tablespoons coconut oil
- 3 cloves of garlic, minced
- 1 onion, chopped
- 1 bunch kale, stems removed and leaves chopped
- 5 white button mushrooms, chopped
- 1 cup of coconut milk
- Salt and pepper to taste

DIRECTIONS:

1. Heat oil in a pot. Sauté the garlic and onion until fragrant for 2 minutes. Stir in mushrooms. Season with pepper and salt. Cook for 8 minutes.
2. Stir in kale and coconut milk. Simmer for 5 minutes. Adjust seasoning to taste.

NUTRITION: Calories: 365 Fat: 33.5 g Carbs: 17.9 g Protein: 6 g

64. Tomato Dill Cauliflower

Preparation time: 15 minutes

Cooking time: 0 minutes

Servings: 4

INGREDIENTS:

- 1 lb. cauliflower florets, chopped
- 1 tablespoon fresh dill, chopped
- ¼ teaspoon Italian seasoning
- 1 tablespoon vinegar
- 1 cup Can tomatoes, crushed
- 1 cup vegetable stock
- 1 teaspoon garlic, minced
- Pepper
- Salt

DIRECTIONS:

1. Add all ingredients except dill into the instant pot and stir well. Seal pot with lid and cook on high for 12 minutes.
2. Once done, allow to release pressure naturally for 10 minutes then release remaining using quick release. Remove lid. Garnish with dill and serve.

NUTRITION: Calories: 47 Fat: 0.3 g Carbs: 10 g Protein: 3.1 g

65. Sautéed Dark Leafy Greens

Preparation time: 15 minutes

Cooking time: 10 minutes

Servings: 4

INGREDIENTS:

- 2 tablespoons olive oil
- 8 cups stemmed and coarsely chopped spinach, kale, collard greens, or Swiss chard
- Juice of ½ lemon
- Sea salt
- Freshly ground black pepper

DIRECTIONS:

1. In a large skillet, heat the olive oil over medium-high heat. Add the greens and toss with tongs until wilted and tender, 8 to 10 minutes.
2. Remove the skillet from the heat and squeeze in the lemon juice, tossing to coat evenly. Season with salt and pepper and serve.

NUTRITION: Calories: 129 Fat: 7g Carbohydrates: 14g

66. Broiled Tomatoes with Feta

Preparation time: 15 minutes

Cooking time: 8 minutes

Servings: 4

INGREDIENTS:

- 4 large tomatoes, cut in half horizontally
- 1 tablespoon olive oil
- 1 teaspoon minced garlic
- ½ cup crumbled feta cheese
- 1 tablespoon chopped fresh basil
- Sea salt
- Freshly ground black pepper

DIRECTIONS:

1. Preheat the oven to broil. Place the tomato halves, cut-side up, in a 9-by-13-inch baking dish and drizzle them with the olive oil. Rub the garlic into the tomatoes.
2. Broil the tomatoes for about 5 minutes, until softened. Sprinkle with the feta cheese and broil for 3 minutes longer. Sprinkle with basil and season with salt and pepper. Serve.

NUTRITION: Calories: 113 Fat: 8g Carbohydrates: 8g Protein: 4g

67. Parmesan-Sautéed Zucchini with Spaghetti

Preparation time: 15 minutes

Cooking time: 15 minutes

Servings: 4

INGREDIENTS:

- 8 ounces dry whole-grain spaghetti
- 2 tablespoons olive oil
- 1 tablespoon minced garlic
- 4 zucchinis, chopped
- ½ cup grated Parmesan cheese, divided
- Sea salt
- Freshly ground black pepper

DIRECTIONS:

1. Bring a large pot of water to a boil and cook the pasta according to the package instructions until al dente. Drain.

2. While the pasta is cooking, in a large skillet, heat the olive oil over medium-high heat. Sauté the garlic until softened, about 2 minutes.

3. Add the zucchini and sauté until the squash is lightly caramelized, about 5 minutes. Stir in ¼ cup of Parmesan cheese and toss until the cheese is melted and lightly browned.

4. Add the cooked spaghetti to the skillet and toss to coat. Season with salt and pepper and serve topped with the remaining ¼ cup of Parmesan cheese.

NUTRITION: Calories: 338 Fat: 11g Carbohydrates: 50g Protein: 15g

68. Wild Rice with Grapes

Preparation time: 15 minutes

Cooking time: 50 minutes

Servings: 4

INGREDIENTS:

- 1 cup wild rice blend
- 1¾ cups water
- 1 teaspoon olive oil
- 2 cups red seedless grapes
- 2 teaspoons chopped fresh thyme
- Sea salt
- Freshly ground black pepper

DIRECTIONS:

1. In a pot, combine the rice and water and bring to a boil. Cover, reduce the heat to low, and simmer for 45 minutes. Remove from the heat and let stand, covered, for 10 minutes. Fluff with a fork.

2. In a large skillet, heat the olive oil over medium-high heat. Add the grapes and thyme and sauté until the grapes begin to burst, about 5 minutes. Stir in the wild rice mixture and season with salt and pepper. Serve.

NUTRITION: Calories: 146 Fat: 2g Carbohydrates: 31g Protein: 3g

69. Traditional Falafel

Preparation time: 15 minutes

Cooking time: 10 minutes

Servings: 4

INGREDIENTS:

- 1 (15-ounce) can low-sodium chickpeas, drained and rinsed
- ½ sweet onion, chopped
- ¼ cup whole-wheat flour
- ¼ cup coarsely chopped fresh parsley
- ¼ cup coarsely chopped fresh cilantro
- Juice from 1 lemon
- 1 tablespoon minced garlic
- 2 teaspoon ground cumin
- Sea salt
- Freshly ground black pepper
- 2 tablespoons olive oil

DIRECTIONS:

1. In a food processor, pulse the chickpeas, onion, flour, parsley, cilantro, lemon juice, garlic, and cumin until the mixture just holds together. Season with salt and pepper and mix again.
2. Scoop out about 2 tablespoons of the mixture, roll into a ball, and flatten it out slightly to form a thick patty. Repeat with the remaining chickpea mixture.
3. In a large skillet, heat the olive oil over medium-high heat and pan-fry the patties until golden brown, about 4 minutes per side. Serve alone or stuffed into pita bread.

NUTRITION: Calories: 245 Fat: 9g Carbohydrates: 36g Protein: 7g

70. **Spicy Split Pea Tabbouleh**

Preparation time: 15 minutes

Cooking time: 45 minutes

Servings: 6

INGREDIENTS:

- 1½ cups split peas
- 4 cups water
- 2 large tomatoes, seeded and chopped
- 1 English cucumber, chopped
- 1 yellow bell pepper, chopped
- 1 orange bell pepper, chopped
- ½ red onion, finely chopped
- ¼ cup chopped fresh cilantro
- Juice of 1 lime
- 1 teaspoon ground cumin
- ½ teaspoon ground coriander
- Pinch red pepper flakes
- Sea salt
- Freshly ground black pepper

DIRECTIONS:

1. In a large saucepan, combine the split peas and water over medium-high heat and bring to a boil. Reduce the heat to low

and simmer, uncovered, until the peas are tender, 40 to 45 minutes. Drain the peas and rinse them in cold water to cool.

2. Transfer the peas to a large bowl and add the tomatoes, cucumber, bell peppers, onion, cilantro, lime juice, cumin, coriander, and red pepper flakes. Toss to mix well.

3. Place the mixture in the refrigerator for at least 1 hour to let the flavors mesh. Season with salt and pepper and serve.

NUTRITION: Calories: 208 Fat: 1g Carbohydrates: 38g Protein: 14g

71. <u>Mashed Avocado Egg Salad with Crisps</u>

Preparation time: 15 minutes

Cooking time: 0 minutes

Servings: 4

INGREDIENTS:

- 6 hard-boiled eggs, peeled and coarsely chopped
- 1 avocado, peeled and pitted
- 1 celery stalk, chopped
- Juice and zest of ½ lemon
- 1 teaspoon chopped fresh parsley
- 4 whole-wheat bread slices, toasted
- 2 tomatoes, thinly sliced
- Sea salt
- Freshly ground black pepper

DIRECTIONS:

1. In a medium bowl, mash the eggs and avocado until well blended but still chunky. Stir in the celery, lemon juice, lemon zest, and parsley until well mixed.

2. Generously spread the egg mixture on the toast and arrange the tomato slices on top. Season with salt and pepper and serve.

NUTRITION: Calories: 248 Fat: 14g Carbohydrates: 18g Protein: 13g

RICE, BEAN, GRAIN

RECIPES

72. Farro Salad Mix

Preparation time: 15 minutes

Cooking time: 33 minutes

Servings: 4-6

INGREDIENTS:

- 1 teaspoon Dijon mustard
- 1½ cups whole farro
- 2 ounces feta cheese, crumbled (½ cup)
- 2 tablespoons lemon juice
- 2 tablespoons minced shallot
- 3 tablespoons chopped fresh dill
- 3 tablespoons extra-virgin olive oil
- 6 ounces asparagus, trimmed and cut into 1-inch lengths
- 6 ounces cherry tomatoes, halved
- 6 ounces sugar snap peas, strings removed, cut into 1-inch lengths
- Salt and pepper

DIRECTIONS:

1. Bring 4 quarts water to boil in a Dutch oven. Put in asparagus, snap peas, and 1 tablespoon salt and cook until crisp-tender, approximately 3 minutes.

2. Use a slotted spoon to move vegetables to large plate and allow to cool completely, about 15 minutes. Put in farro to water, return to boil, and cook until grains are soft with slight chew, 15 to 30 minutes.

3. Drain farro, spread in rimmed baking sheet, and allow to cool completely, about 15 minutes.

4. Beat oil, lemon juice, shallot, mustard, ¼ teaspoon salt, and ¼ teaspoon pepper together in a big container.

5. Put in vegetables, farro, tomatoes, dill, and ¼ cup feta and toss gently to combine. Sprinkle with salt and pepper to taste. Move to serving platter and drizzle with remaining ¼ cup feta. Serve.

NUTRITION: Calories: 240 Carbs: 26g Fat: 12g Protein: 9g

73. Farrotto Mix

Preparation time: 15 minutes

Cooking time: 40 minutes

Servings: 6

INGREDIENTS:

- ½ onion, chopped fine
- 1 cup frozen peas, thawed

- 1 garlic clove, minced

- 1 tablespoon minced fresh chives

- 1 teaspoon grated lemon zest plus 1 teaspoon juice

- 1½ cups whole farro

- 1½ ounces Parmesan cheese, grated (¾ cup)

- 2 tablespoons extra-virgin olive oil

- 2 teaspoons minced fresh tarragon

- 3 cups chicken broth

- 3 cups water

- 4 ounces asparagus, trimmed and cut on bias into 1-inch lengths

- 4 ounces pancetta, cut into ¼-inch pieces

- Salt and pepper

DIRECTIONS:

1. Pulse farro using a blender until about half of grains are broken into smaller pieces, about 6 pulses.

2. Bring broth and water to boil in moderate-sized saucepan on high heat. Put in asparagus and cook until crisp-tender, 2 to 3 minutes.

3. Use a slotted spoon to move asparagus to a container and set aside. Decrease heat to low, cover broth mixture, and keep warm.

4. Cook pancetta in a Dutch oven on moderate heat until lightly browned and fat has rendered, approximately 5 minutes.

5. Put in 1 tablespoon oil and onion and cook till they become tender, approximately 5 minutes. Mix in garlic and cook until aromatic, approximately half a minute.

6. Put in farro and cook, stirring often, until grains are lightly toasted, approximately three minutes.

7. Stir 5 cups warm broth mixture into farro mixture, decrease the heat to low, cover, and cook until almost all liquid has been absorbed and farro is just al dente, about 25 minutes, stirring twice during cooking.

8. Put in peas, tarragon, ¾ teaspoon salt, and ½ teaspoon pepper and cook, stirring continuously, until farro becomes creamy, approximately 5 minutes.

9. Remove from the heat, mix in Parmesan, chives, lemon zest and juice, remaining 1 tablespoon oil, and reserved asparagus.

10. Adjust consistency with remaining warm broth mixture as required (you may have broth left over). Sprinkle with salt and pepper to taste. Serve.

NUTRITION: Calories: 218 Carbs: 41g Fat: 2g Protein: 7g

74. Fennel-Parmesan Farro

Preparation time: 15 minutes

Cooking time: 50 minutes

Servings: 4-6

INGREDIENTS:

- ¼ cup minced fresh parsley

- 1 onion, chopped fine
- 1 ounce Parmesan cheese, grated (½ cup)
- 1 small fennel bulb, stalks discarded, bulb halved, cored, and chopped fine
- 1 teaspoon minced fresh thyme or ¼ teaspoon dried
- 1½ cups whole farro
- 2 teaspoons sherry vinegar
- 3 garlic cloves, minced
- 3 tablespoons extra-virgin olive oil
- Salt and pepper

DIRECTIONS:

1. Bring 4 quarts water to boil in a Dutch oven. Put in farro and 1 tablespoon salt, return to boil, and cook until grains are soft with slight chew, 15 to 30 minutes.

2. Drain farro, return to now-empty pot, and cover to keep warm. Heat 2 tablespoons oil in 12-inch frying pan on moderate heat until it starts to shimmer.

3. Put in onion, fennel, and ¼ teaspoon salt and cook, stirring intermittently, till they become tender, 8 to 10 minutes. Put in garlic and thyme and cook until aromatic, approximately half a minute.

4. Put in residual 1 tablespoon oil and farro and cook, stirring often, until heated through, approximately 2 minutes.

5. Remove from the heat, mix in Parmesan, parsley, and vinegar. Sprinkle with salt and pepper to taste. Serve.

NUTRITION: Calories: 338 Carbs: 56g Fat: 10g Protein: 11g

75. Feta-Grape-Bulgur Salad with Grapes and Feta

Preparation time: 15 minutes

Cooking time: 1 hour & 30 minutes

Servings: 4-6

INGREDIENTS:

- ¼ cup chopped fresh mint
- ¼ cup extra-virgin olive oil
- ¼ teaspoon ground cumin
- ½ cup slivered almonds, toasted
- 1 cup water
- 1½ cups medium-grind bulgur, rinsed
- 2 ounces feta cheese, crumbled (½ cup)
- 2 scallions, sliced thin
- 5 tablespoons lemon juice (2 lemons)
- 6 ounces seedless red grapes, quartered (1 cup)
- Pinch cayenne pepper
- Salt and pepper

DIRECTIONS:

1. Mix bulgur, water, ¼ cup lemon juice, and ¼ teaspoon salt in a container. Cover and allow to sit at room temperature until grains are softened and liquid is fully absorbed, about 1½ hours.

2. Beat remaining 1 tablespoon lemon juice, oil, cumin, cayenne, and ¼ teaspoon salt together in a big container.

3. Put in bulgur, grapes, 1/3 cup almonds, 1/3 cup feta, scallions, and mint and gently toss to combine. Sprinkle with salt and pepper to taste. Sprinkle with remaining almonds and remaining feta before you serve.

NUTRITION: Calories: 500 Carbs: 45g Fat: 14g Protein: 50g

76. Greek Style Meaty Bulgur

Preparation time: 15 minutes

Cooking time: 30 minutes

Servings: 4-6

INGREDIENTS:

- ½ cup jarred roasted red peppers, rinsed, patted dry, and chopped
- 1 bay leaf
- 1 cup medium-grind bulgur, rinsed
- 1 onion, chopped fine
- 1 tablespoon chopped fresh dill
- 1 teaspoon extra-virgin olive oil
- 1 1/3 cups vegetable broth

- 2 teaspoons minced fresh marjoram or ½ teaspoon dried
- 3 garlic cloves, minced
- 8 ounces ground lamb
- Lemon wedges
- Salt and pepper

DIRECTIONS:

1. Heat oil in a big saucepan on moderate to high heat until just smoking. Put in lamb, ½ teaspoon salt, and ¼ teaspoon pepper and cook, breaking up meat with wooden spoon, until browned, 3 to 5 minutes.

2. Mix in onion and red peppers and cook until onion is softened, 5 to 7 minutes. Mix in garlic and marjoram and cook until aromatic, approximately half a minute.

3. Mix in bulgur, broth, and bay leaf and bring to simmer. Decrease heat to low, cover, and simmer gently until bulgur is tender, 16 to 18 minutes.

4. Remove from the heat, lay clean dish towel underneath lid and let bulgur sit for about 10 minutes.

5. Put in dill and fluff gently with fork to combine. Sprinkle with salt and pepper to taste. Serve with lemon wedges.

NUTRITION: Calories: 137 Carbs: 16g Fat: 5g Protein: 7g

77. Hearty Barley Mix

Preparation time: 15 minutes

Cooking time: 50 minutes

Servings: 4

INGREDIENTS:

- 1/8 teaspoon ground cardamom
- ½ cup plain yogurt
- ½ teaspoon ground cumin
- 2/3 cup raw sunflower seeds
- ¾ teaspoon ground coriander
- 1 cup pearl barley
- 1½ tablespoons minced fresh mint
- 1½ teaspoons grated lemon zest plus 1½ tablespoons juice
- 3 tablespoons extra-virgin olive oil
- 5 carrots, peeled
- 8 ounces snow peas, strings removed, halved along the length
- Salt and pepper

DIRECTIONS:

1. Beat yogurt, ½ teaspoon lemon zest and 1½ teaspoons juice, 1½ teaspoons mint, ¼ teaspoon salt, and 1/8 teaspoon pepper together in a small-sized container; cover put inside your fridge until ready to serve.

2. Bring 4 quarts water to boil in a Dutch oven. Put in barley and 1 tablespoon salt, return to boil, and cook until tender, 20 to 40 minutes. Drain barley, return to now-empty pot, and cover to keep warm.

3. In the meantime, halve carrots crosswise, then halve or quarter along the length to create uniformly sized pieces.

4. Heat 1 tablespoon oil in 12-inch frying pan on moderate to high heat until just smoking. Put in carrots and ½ teaspoon coriander and cook, stirring intermittently, until mildly charred and just tender, 5 to 7 minutes.

5. Put in snow peas and cook, stirring intermittently, until spotty brown, 3 to 5 minutes; move to plate.

6. Heat 1½ teaspoons oil in now-empty frying pan on moderate heat until it starts to shimmer. Put in sunflower seeds, cumin, cardamom, remaining ¼ teaspoon coriander, and ¼ teaspoon salt.

7. Cook, stirring continuously, until seeds are toasted, approximately 2 minutes; move to small-sized container.

8. Beat remaining 1 teaspoon lemon zest and 1 tablespoon juice, remaining 1 tablespoon mint, and remaining 1½ tablespoons oil together in a big container.

9. Put in barley and carrot–snow pea mixture and gently toss to combine. Sprinkle with salt and pepper to taste. Serve, topping individual portions with spiced sunflower seeds and drizzling with yogurt sauce.

NUTRITION: Calories: 193 Carbs: 44g Fat: 1g Protein: 4g

78. Hearty Barley Risotto

Preparation time: 15 minutes

Cooking time: 60 minutes

Servings: 4-6

INGREDIENTS:

- 1 carrot, peeled and chopped fine
- 1 cup dry white wine
- 1 onion, chopped fine
- 1 teaspoon minced fresh thyme or ¼ teaspoon dried
- 1½ cups pearl barley
- 2 ounces Parmesan cheese, grated (1 cup)
- 2 tablespoons extra-virgin olive oil
- 4 cups chicken or vegetable broth
- 4 cups water
- Salt and pepper

DIRECTIONS:

1. Bring broth and water to simmer in moderate-sized saucepan. Decrease heat to low and cover to keep warm.

2. Heat 1 tablespoon oil in a Dutch oven on moderate heat until it starts to shimmer. Put in onion and carrot and cook till they become tender, 5 to 7 minutes.

3. Put in barley and cook, stirring frequently, until lightly toasted and aromatic, about 4 minutes. Put in wine and cook, stirring often, until fully absorbed, approximately two minutes.

4. Mix in 3 cups warm broth and thyme, bring to simmer, and cook, stirring intermittently, until liquid is absorbed and bottom of pot is dry, 22 to 25 minutes.

5. Mix in 2 cups warm broth, bring to simmer, and cook, stirring intermittently, until liquid is absorbed and bottom of pot is dry, fifteen to twenty minutes.

6. Carry on cooking risotto, stirring frequently and adding warm broth as required to stop pot bottom from becoming dry, until barley is cooked through, 15 to 20 minutes.

7. Remove from the heat, adjust consistency with remaining warm broth as required. Mix in Parmesan and residual 1 tablespoon oil and sprinkle with salt and pepper to taste. Serve.

NUTRITION: Calories: 222 Carbs: 33g Fat: 5g Protein: 6g

79. Hearty Freekeh Pilaf

Preparation time: 15 minutes

Cooking time: 60 minutes

Servings: 4-6

INGREDIENTS:

- ¼ cup chopped fresh mint
- ¼ cup extra-virgin olive oil, plus extra for serving
- ¼ cup shelled pistachios, toasted and coarsely chopped
- ¼ teaspoon ground coriander
- ¼ teaspoon ground cumin
- 1 head cauliflower (2 pounds), cored and cut into ½-inch florets
- 1 shallot, minced
- 1½ cups whole freekeh

- 1½ tablespoons lemon juice
- 1½ teaspoons grated fresh ginger
- 3 ounces pitted dates, chopped (½ cup)
- Salt and pepper

DIRECTIONS:

1. Bring 4 quarts water to boil in a Dutch oven. Put in freekeh and 1 tablespoon salt, return to boil, and cook until grains are tender, 30 to 45 minutes. Drain freekeh, return to now-empty pot, and cover to keep warm.

2. Heat 2 tablespoons oil in 12-inch non-stick frying pan on moderate to high heat until it starts to shimmer.

3. Put in cauliflower, ½ teaspoon salt, and ¼ teaspoon pepper, cover, and cook until florets are softened and start to brown, approximately five minutes.

4. Remove lid and continue to cook, stirring intermittently, until florets turn spotty brown, about 10 minutes.

5. Put in remaining 2 tablespoons oil, dates, shallot, ginger, coriander, and cumin and cook, stirring often, until dates and shallot are softened and aromatic, approximately 3 minutes.

6. Decrease heat to low, put in freekeh, and cook, stirring often, until heated through, about 1 minute. Remove from the heat, mix in pistachios, mint, and lemon juice.

7. Sprinkle with salt and pepper to taste and drizzle with extra oil. Serve.

NUTRITION: Calories: 520 Carbs: 54g Fat: 14g Protein: 36g

80. Herby-Lemony Farro

Preparation time: 15 minutes

Cooking time: 40 minutes

Servings: 4-6

INGREDIENTS:

- ¼ cup chopped fresh mint
- ¼ cup chopped fresh parsley
- 1 garlic clove, minced
- 1 onion, chopped fine
- 1 tablespoon lemon juice
- 1½ cups whole farro
- 3 tablespoons extra-virgin olive oil
- Salt and pepper

DIRECTIONS:

1. Bring 4 quarts water to boil in a Dutch oven. Put in farro and 1 tablespoon salt, return to boil, and cook until grains are soft with slight chew, 15 to 30 minutes. Drain farro, return to now-empty pot, and cover to keep warm.

2. Heat 2 tablespoons oil in 12-inch frying pan on moderate heat until it starts to shimmer. Put in onion and ¼ teaspoon salt and cook till they become tender, approximately five minutes.

3. Mix in garlic and cook until aromatic, approximately half a minute. Put in residual 1 tablespoon oil and farro and cook, stirring often, until heated through, approximately two minutes.

4. Remove from the heat, mix in parsley, mint, and lemon juice. Sprinkle with salt and pepper to taste. Serve.

NUTRITION: Calories: 243 Carbs: 22g Fat: 14g Protein: 10g

81. Mushroom-Bulgur Pilaf

Preparation time: 15 minutes

Cooking time: 30 minutes

Servings: 4

INGREDIENTS:

- ¼ cup minced fresh parsley
- ¼ ounce dried porcini mushrooms, rinsed and minced
- ¾ cup chicken or vegetable broth
- ¾ cup water
- 1 cup medium-grind bulgur, rinsed
- 1 onion, chopped fine
- 2 garlic cloves, minced
- 2 tablespoons extra-virgin olive oil
- 8 ounces cremini mushrooms, trimmed, halved if small or quartered if large
- Salt and pepper

DIRECTIONS:

1. Heat oil in a big saucepan on moderate heat until it starts to shimmer. Put in onion, porcini mushrooms, and ½ teaspoon salt and cook until onion is softened, approximately 5 minutes.

2. Mix in cremini mushrooms, increase heat to medium-high, cover, and cook until cremini release their liquid and begin to brown, about 4 minutes.

3. Mix in garlic and cook until aromatic, approximately half a minute. Mix in bulgur, broth, and water and bring to simmer.

4. Decrease heat to low, cover, and simmer gently until bulgur is tender, 16 to 18 minutes. Remove from the heat, lay clean dish towel underneath lid and let pilaf sit for about ten minutes.

5. Put in parsley to pilaf and fluff gently with fork to combine. Sprinkle with salt and pepper to taste. Serve.

NUTRITION: Calories: 259 Carbs: 50g Fat: 3g Protein: 11g

PASTA RECIPES

82. Pasta Fazool (Pasta e Fagioli)

Preparation time: 15 minutes

Cooking time: 25 minutes

Servings: 2

INGREDIENTS:

- 1 tablespoon of olive oil,
- 12 ounces of Italian sweet bulk sausage
- 1 celery stem, diced
- 1/2 yellow onion, chopped
- 3/4 cup dry macaroni
- 1/4 cup tomato puree
- 3 cups chicken broth or more if necessary, divided
- salt and freshly ground black pepper
- 1/4 teaspoon of ground red pepper flakes
- 1/4 teaspoon dried oregano
- 3 cups finely chopped chard
- 1 can cannellini (15 oz), drained
- 1/4 cup grated Parmigiano-Reggiano cheese

DIRECTIONS:

1. Heat the oil in a frying pan over medium heat. Brown the sausage by cutting it into small pieces, about 5 minutes. Return the heat to medium.

2. Add diced celery and chopped onion. Bake until the onions are transparent, 4 to 5 minutes. Add the dry pasta. Boil and stir for 2 minutes.

3. Stir the tomato puree until smooth, 2 to 3 minutes. Add 3 cups of broth. Turn up the heat and let it simmer. Season with salt, black pepper, pepper flakes, and oregano.

4. Lower heat once soup comes to a boil, then let it simmer for about 5 minutes, often stirring. Check the consistency of the soup and add stock if necessary.

5. Place the chopped chard in a bowl. And soak with cold water to rinse the leaves; some grain will fall to the bottom of the bowl.

6. Transfer the chard to a colander to drain briefly; add to the soup. Boil and stir until the leaves fade, 2 to 3 minutes.

7. Stir in the white beans; keep cooking, stir until the pasta is cooked, 4 or 5 minutes. Remove from heat and stir in the grated cheese. Serve garnished with grated cheese, if desired.

NUTRITION: Calories 888 Fat 43.8 g Carbohydrates 77.3 g Protein 43.8 g

83. Pasta Orecchiette Pasta

Preparation time: 15 minutes

Cooking time: 28 minutes

Servings: 2

INGREDIENTS:

- 2 tablespoons olive oil
- 1/2 onion, salt, diced to taste
- 8 grams of spicy Italian sausage
- 3 1/2 cups low-sodium chicken broth, divided
- 1 1/4 cup orecchiette pasta
- 1/2 cup of arugula
- 1/4 cup finely grated Parmigiano-Reggiano cheese

DIRECTIONS:

1. Heat the olive oil in a deep-frying pan over medium heat. Cook and stir the onion with a pinch of salt in hot oil until the onion is soft and golden brown, 5 to 7 minutes.
2. Stir the sausages with onions; cook and stir until the sausages are golden brown, 5 to 7 minutes. Pour 1 1/2 cup chicken stock into the sausage mixture and bring to a boil.
3. Add the pasta to the orecchiette; boil and mix the pasta in a warm broth, add the remaining broth when the liquid is absorbed until the pasta is well cooked, and most of the broth is absorbed, about 15 minutes.
4. Spread the pasta in bowls and sprinkle with Parmigiano-Reggiano cheese.

NUTRITION: Calories 662 Fat 39.1 g Carbohydrates 46.2 g Protein 31.2 g

84. Shrimp Scampi with Pasta

Preparation time: 15 minutes

Cooking time: 20 minutes

Servings: 6

INGREDIENTS:

- 1 pack of linguine (16 oz)
- 2 tablespoons butter
- 2 tablespoons extra virgin olive oil
- 2 chopped shallots
- 2 cloves of chopped garlic
- 1 pinch of red pepper flakes
- 1 pound of shrimp, peeled and thawed
- 1 pinch of kosher salt and freshly ground pepper
- 1/2 cup of dry white wine
- 1 lemon, juiced
- 2 tablespoons butter
- 2 tablespoons extra virgin olive oil
- 1/4 cup finely chopped fresh parsley leaves
- 1 teaspoon extra virgin olive oil

DIRECTIONS:

1. Boil a large pot of salted water to a boil; Add linguine in boiling water for 6 to 8 minutes until soft. Drain.

2. Melt 2 tablespoons of butter in a large frying pan followed by 2 tablespoons of olive oil over medium-high heat.

3. Lightly fry the shallots, garlic, and red pepper flakes in the hot butter and oil until the shallots are transparent, 3 to 4 minutes.

4. Season the shrimp with kosher salt and black pepper; Add to the pan and cook until pink, occasionally stirring, 2 to 3 minutes. Remove the shrimp from the pan and keep them warm.

5. Pour the white wine and lemon juice into the pan and bring to a boil. Melt 2 tablespoons of butter in a pan, mix 2 tablespoons of olive oil and let it simmer.

6. Mix the linguine, shrimp, and parsley in the butter mixture until everything is well covered; Season with salt and black pepper. Sprinkle with 1 teaspoon of olive oil to serve.

NUTRITION: Calories 511 Fat 19.4 g Carbohydrates 57.5 g Protein 21.9 g

85. **Pasta Salad with Chicken Club**

Preparation time: 15 minutes

Cooking time: 12 minutes

Servings: 6

INGREDIENTS:

- 8 oz corkscrew pasta
- 3/4 cup Italian dressing
- 1/4 cup mayonnaise
- 2 cups roasted chicken cooked and minced

- 12 slices of crispy cooked bacon, crumbled
- 1 cup diced Münster cheese
- 1 cup chopped celery
- 1 cup chopped green pepper
- 8 oz. Cherry tomatoes, halved
- 1 avocado - peeled, seeded and chopped

DIRECTIONS:

1. Bring a large pan of lightly salted water to a boil. Boil the pasta, occasionally stirring until well-cooked but firm, 10 to 12 minutes. Drain and rinse with cold water.

2. Beat the Italian dressing and mayonnaise in a large bowl. Stir the pasta, chicken, bacon, Münster cheese, celery, green pepper, cherry tomatoes, and avocado through the vinaigrette until everything is well mixed.

NUTRITION: Calories 485 Fat 30.1 g Carbohydrates 37.1 g Protein 19.2 g

86. Sausage Pasta

Preparation time: 15 minutes

Cooking time: 20 minutes

Servings: 6

INGREDIENTS:

- 3/4 pound of pasta
- 1 tablespoon of olive oil

- Spicy Italian sausage of 1 pound
- 1 onion, minced
- 4 cloves of chopped garlic
- 1 canned chicken broth
- 1 teaspoon dried basil
- 1 can diced tomatoes
- 1 pack (10 oz) of frozen chopped spinach
- 1/2 cup of grated Parmesan cheese

DIRECTIONS:

1. Boil lightly salted water in a large pot, then add pasta and cook until al dente; (8-10 minutes). Drain and set aside.
2. Heat oil and sausage in a large skillet; cook until pink. Add the onion and garlic to the pan during the last 5 minutes of cooking. Add the stock, basil, and tomatoes with the liquid.
3. Simmer over medium heat for 5 minutes to reduce slightly. Add the chopped spinach; cover the pan and simmer over low heat until the spinach is soft.
4. Add the pasta to the pan and mix. Sprinkle with cheese and serve immediately.

NUTRITION: Calories 423 Fat 19.3 g Carbohydrates 39 g Protein 22.3 g

87. Pomodoro Pasta

Preparation time: 15 minutes

Cooking time: 25 minutes

Servings: 4

INGREDIENTS:

- 1 pack of 16 angel hair pasta
- 1/4 cup of olive oil
- 1/2 onion, minced
- 4 cloves of chopped garlic
- 2 cups of Roma tomatoes, diced
- 2 tablespoons balsamic vinegar
- 1 low-sodium chicken broth
- ground red pepper
- freshly ground black pepper to taste
- 1/4 cup grated Parmesan cheese
- 2 tablespoons chopped fresh basil

DIRECTIONS:

1. Bring a large pot of lightly salted water to a boil. Add pasta and cook for 8 minutes or until al dente; drain.

2. Pour the olive oil in a large deep pan over high heat. Fry onions and garlic until light brown. Lower the heat to medium and add tomatoes, vinegar, and chicken stock; simmer for about 8 minutes.

3. Stir in the red pepper, black pepper, basil, and cooked pasta and mix well with the sauce. Simmer for about 5 minutes and serve garnished with grated cheese.

NUTRITION: Calories 500 Fat 18.3 g Carbohydrates 69.7 g Protein 16.2 g

88. Fra Diavolo Pasta Sauce

Preparation time: 15 minutes

Cooking time: 55 minutes

Servings: 8

INGREDIENTS:

- 4 tablespoons olive oil, divided
- 6 cloves of garlic, crushed
- 3 cups peeled whole tomatoes with liquid, chopped
- 1 1/2 teaspoon of salt
- 1 teaspoon crushed red pepper flakes
- 1 packet of linguine pasta
- 8 grams of small shrimp, peeled
- 8 grams of bay scallops
- 1 tablespoon of chopped fresh parsley

DIRECTIONS:

1. Heat 2 tablespoons of olive oil and sauté garlic over medium heat. When the garlic starts to sizzle, pour in the tomatoes.
2. Season with salt and red pepper. Bring to boil. Reduce the heat and simmer for 30 minutes, stirring occasionally.
3. Meanwhile, boil a large pan with lightly salted water. Cook pasta for about 8 to 10 minutes or until al dente; drain.

4. Heat the remaining 2 tablespoons of olive oil in a large frying pan over high heat. Add shrimps and scallops. Cook for about 2 minutes stirring regularly, or until the shrimp turn pink.

5. Add the shrimp and scallops to the tomato mixture and stir in the parsley. Bake for 3 to 4 minutes or until the sauce starts to bubble. Serve the sauce on the pasta.

NUTRITION: Calories 335 Fat 8.9 g Carbohydrates 46.3 g Protein 18.7 g

89. Ranch Bacon Pasta Salad

Preparation time: 15 minutes

Cooking time: 15 minutes

Servings: 10

INGREDIENTS:

- 1 (12 oz.) package of uncooked tri color rotini
- 10 slices of bacon
- 1 cup mayonnaise
- 3 tablespoons dry ranch dressing powder
- 1/4 teaspoon of garlic powder
- 1/2 teaspoon of garlic pepper
- 1/2 cup of milk
- 1 large tomato, minced
- 1 can of sliced black olives (4.25 oz)
- 1 cup grated cheddar cheese

DIRECTIONS:

1. Bring a large pot of lightly salted water to a boil; cook the rotini until tender but firm, about 8 minutes; drain.

2. Place the bacon in a frying pan over medium heat and cook until evenly browned. Drain and chop.

3. Combine mayonnaise, ranch dressing, garlic powder, and garlic pepper in a large bowl. Stir the milk until smooth.

4. Put the rotini, bacon, tomatoes, black olives, and cheese in a bowl and mix to cover with vinaigrette. Cover and put in the fridge for at least 1 hour.

NUTRITION: Calories 336 Fat 26.8 g Carbohydrates 14.9 g Protein 9.3 g

90. Alfredo Peppered Shrimp

Preparation time: 15 minutes

Cooking time: 20 minutes

Servings: 6

INGREDIENTS:

- 3 pounds penne
- 1/4 cup butter
- 2 tablespoons extra virgin olive oil
- 1 onion, diced
- 2 cloves of chopped garlic
- 1 red pepper, diced

- 1-pound portobello mushrooms, cubed
- 1 pound shrimp, peeled and thawed
- 1 jar of Alfredo sauce
- 1/2 cup of grated Romano cheese
- 1/2 cup of cream
- 1/4 cup chopped parsley
- 1 teaspoon cayenne pepper
- salt and pepper to taste

DIRECTIONS:

1. Bring a large pot of lightly salted water to a boil. Put the pasta and cook for 8 to 10 minutes or until al dente; drain.
2. Meanwhile, melt the butter and olive oil in a pan over medium heat. Stir in the onion and cook until soft and translucent, about 2 minutes.
3. Stir in garlic, red pepper and mushrooms; cook over medium heat until soft, about 2 minutes longer.
4. Stir in the shrimp and fry until firm and pink, then add Alfredo sauce, Romano cheese and cream; bring to a boil, constantly stirring until thick, about 5 minutes.
5. Season with cayenne pepper, salt, and pepper to taste. Add the drained pasta to the sauce and sprinkle with chopped parsley.

NUTRITION: Calories 707 Fat 45 g Carbohydrates 50.6 g Protein 28.4 g

91. Bow Ties with Sausages, Tomatoes & Cream

Preparation time: 15 minutes

Cooking time: 25 minutes

Servings: 6

INGREDIENTS:

- 1 package of bowtie pasta
- 2 tablespoons of olive oil
- 1 pound of sweet Italian sausages, crumbled
- 1/2 teaspoon of red pepper flakes
- 1/2 cup diced onion
- 3 finely chopped garlic cloves
- 1 can of Italian tomatoes, drained and roughly chopped
- 1 1/2 cup whipped cream
- 1/2 teaspoon salt
- 3 tablespoons fresh parsley

DIRECTIONS:

1. Bring a large pot of lightly salted water to a boil. Cook the pasta for 8 to 10 minutes in boiling water or until al dente; drain.
2. Heat the oil in a deep-frying pan over medium heat. Cook the sausages and chili flakes until the sausages are golden brown.

3. Stir in onion and garlic and cook until the onion is soft. Stir in the tomatoes, cream, and salt. Simmer until thickened, 8 to 10 minutes.

4. Add the pasta cooked in the sauce and heat. Sprinkle with parsley.

NUTRITION: Calories 656 Fat 42.1 g Carbohydrates 50.9 g Protein 20.1 g

PIZZA RECIPES

92. Fruit Pizza

Preparation time: 15 minutes

Cooking time: 0 minutes

Servings: 4

INGREDIENTS:

- 4 watermelon slices
- 1 oz blueberries
- 2 oz goat cheese, crumbled
- 1 teaspoon fresh parsley, chopped

DIRECTIONS:

1. Put the watermelon slices in the plate in one layer. Then sprinkle them with blueberries, goat cheese, and fresh parsley.

NUTRITION: Calories 69 Protein 4.4g Carbohydrates 1.4g Fat 5.1g

93. Sprouts Pizza

Preparation time: 15 minutes

Cooking time: 15 minutes

Servings: 6

INGREDIENTS:

- 4 oz wheat flour, whole grain
- 2 tablespoons olive oil
- ¼ teaspoon baking powder
- 5 oz chicken fillet, boiled
- 2 oz Mozzarella cheese, shredded
- 1 tomato, chopped
- 2 oz bean sprouts

DIRECTIONS:

1. Make the pizza crust: mix wheat flour, olive oil, baking powder, and knead the dough. Roll it up in the shape of pizza crust and transfer in the pizza mold.

2. Then sprinkle it with chopped tomato, shredded chicken, and Mozzarella. Bake the pizza at 365F for 15 minutes. Sprinkle the cooked pizza with bean sprouts and cut into servings.

NUTRITION: Calories 184 Protein 11.9g Carbohydrates 15.6g Fat 8.2g

94. **Cheese Pinwheels**

Preparation time: 15 minutes

Cooking time: 25 minutes

Servings: 6

INGREDIENTS:

- 1 teaspoon chili flakes
- ½ teaspoon dried cilantro

- 1 egg, beaten
- 1 teaspoon cream cheese
- 1 oz Cheddar cheese, grated
- 6 oz pizza dough

DIRECTIONS:

1. Roll up the pizza dough and cut into 6 squares. Sprinkle the dough with dried cilantro, cream cheese, and Cheddar cheese.
2. Roll the dough in the shape of pinwheels, brush with beaten egg and bake in the preheated to 365F oven for 25 minutes or until the pinwheels are light brown.

NUTRITION: Calories 16 Protein 3.8g Carbohydrates 12.1g Fat 11.2g

95. Ground Meat Pizza

Preparation time: 15 minutes

Cooking time: 35 minutes

Servings: 4

INGREDIENTS:

- 7 oz ground beef
- 1 teaspoon tomato paste
- ½ teaspoon ground black pepper
- 2 egg whites, whisked
- ½ cup Mozzarella cheese, shredded
- 1 teaspoon fresh basil, chopped

DIRECTIONS:

1. Line the baking tray with baking paper. Preheat the oven to 370F. Mix all ingredients except Mozzarella in the mixing bowl.

2. Then place the mixture in the tray and flatten it to get a thick layer. Top the pizza with Mozzarella cheese and bake in the oven for 35 minutes. Then cut the cooked pizza into the servings.

NUTRITION: Calories 113 Protein 18g Carbohydrates 0.7g Fat 3.8g

96. Quinoa Flour Pizza

Preparation time: 15 minutes

Cooking time: 15 minutes

Servings: 6

INGREDIENTS:

- 1 oz pumpkin puree
- 3 tablespoons quinoa flour
- ½ teaspoon dried oregano
- 1 cup Mozzarella cheese, shredded
- 1 tomato, chopped
- 1 teaspoon olive oil

DIRECTIONS:

1. Mix pumpkin puree, quinoa flour, and olive oil. Knead the dough. Roll it up in the shape of pizza crust and transfer in the lined with a baking paper baking tray.

2. Then top the pizza crust with tomato, oregano, and Mozzarella cheese. Bake the pizza at 365F for 15 minutes.

NUTRITION: Calories 38 Protein 2g Carbohydrates 3.3g Fat 1.8g

97. Artichoke Pizza

Preparation time: 15 minutes

Cooking time: 20 minutes

Servings: 4

INGREDIENTS:

- 7 oz pizza crust
- 5 oz artichoke hearts, canned, drained, chopped
- 1 teaspoon fresh basil, chopped
- 1 tomato, sliced
- 1 cup Monterey Jack cheese, shredded

DIRECTIONS:

1. Line the pizza mold with baking paper. Then put the pizza crust inside. Top it with sliced tomato, canned artichoke hearts, and basil.
2. Then top the pizza with Monterey Jack cheese and transfer in the preheated to 365F oven. Cook the pizza for 20 minutes.

NUTRITION: Calories 247 Protein 12.1g Carbohydrates 28.2g Fat 10.2g

98. 3-Cheese Pizza

Preparation time: 15 minutes

Cooking time: 10 minutes

Servings: 6

INGREDIENTS:

- 1 pizza crust, cooked
- ½ cup Mozzarella, shredded
- ½ cup Cheddar cheese, shredded
- 2 oz Parmesan, grated
- ¼ cup tomato sauce
- 1 teaspoon Italian seasonings

DIRECTIONS:

1. Put the pizza crust in the baking pan. Then brush it with tomato sauce and Italian seasonings.
2. After this, sprinkle the pizza with Mozzarella, Cheddar cheese, and Parmesan. Bake the pizza for 10 minutes at 375F.

NUTRITION: Calories 106 Protein 7g Carbohydrates 6.3g Fat 6.1g

99. Chickpea Pizza

Preparation time: 15 minutes

Cooking time: 25 minutes

Servings: 6

INGREDIENTS:

- 4 tablespoons marinara sauce
- 7 oz pizza dough
- 1 tomato, sliced
- 1 red onion, sliced
- 5 oz chickpeas, canned
- ½ cup Mozzarella cheese, shredded

DIRECTIONS:

1. Roll up the pizza dough in the shape of pizza crust and transfer in the pizza mold. Then brush the pizza crust with marinara sauce and sprinkle with sliced onion, tomato, and chickpeas.
2. Top the chickpeas with mozzarella cheese and bake the pizza for 25 minutes at 355F.

NUTRITION: Calories 266 Protein 7.6g Carbohydrates 31.9g Fat 12.4g

100. Margherita Pizza

Preparation time: 15 minutes

Cooking time: 15 minutes

Servings: 6

INGREDIENTS:

- 1 pizza crust
- 1 tablespoon olive oil

- 1 cup tomatoes, canned
- 1 cup Mozzarella cheese, shredded
- 1 tablespoon fresh basil leaves

DIRECTIONS:

1. Put the canned tomatoes over the pizza crust, flatten them gently and sprinkle with olive oil. Then top the pizza crust with mozzarella and fresh basil. Bake the pizza at 400F for 15 minutes.

NUTRITION: Calories 94 Protein 3.4g Carbohydrates 12.7g Fat 3.5g

101. Hummus Pizza

Preparation time: 15 minutes

Cooking time: 20 minutes

Servings: 6

INGREDIENTS:

- 6 oz pizza dough
- 5 oz hummus
- 3 oz Feta cheese, crumbled
- 1 tablespoon fresh parsley, chopped
- ½ cup black olives, sliced
- 3 sun-dried tomatoes, chopped
- 1 tablespoon avocado oil

DIRECTIONS:

1. Roll up the pizza dough in the shape of the pizza crust. Then place it in pizza mold and brush with avocado oil.
2. Spread the pizza crust with hummus and sprinkle with parsley, black olives, and sun-dried tomatoes, and crumbled feta. Bake the pizza at 400F for 20 minutes.

NUTRITION: Calories 237 Protein 6.2g Carbohydrates 19.2g Fat 15.6g

CONCLUSION

My utmost gratitude with your support with this book.

As we end here are some more tips to help you with your Mediterranean Diet Journey.

Stay Hydrated

Once you've started and are fully immersed in the Mediterranean diet, you might notice that you've started to feel a little bit week, and a little bit colder, than you're used to. The Mediterranean diet places an emphasis on trying to cut out as much sodium from your diet as possible, which is very healthy for some of us who already have high sodium levels. Sodium, obviously is found in salt, and so we proceed to cut out salt – and then drink enough water to drain every last drop of sodium from our bodies. When it comes to hydration, the biological mechanisms for keeping us saturated and quenched rely on an equal balance of sodium and potassium. Sodium can be found in your interstitial fluid, and potassium can be found inside our cytoplasm – two sides of one wall. When you drink tons of water, sweat a lot at the gym, or both, your sodium leaves your body in your urine and your sweat. Potassium, on the other hand, is only really lost through the urine – and even then, it's rare. This means that our bodies almost constantly need a refill on our sodium levels.

Vitamins and Supplements

Vitamins and minerals can be found in plants and animals, yes, but more often than not fruits and vegetables are much stronger sources. When consume another animal, we are consuming the sum total of all of the energy and nutrition that that animal has also consumed. This might sound like a sweet deal, but the pig you're eating used that energy in his own daily life, and therefore only has a tiny bit left to offer you. Plants, on the other hand, are first-hand sources of things like calcium, vitamin K, and vitamin C, which our bodies require daily doses of.

Meal Preparation and Portion Planning

If you haven't heard of the term "meal prep" before now, it's a beautiful day to learn something that will save you time, stress, and inches on your waistline. Meal prep, short for meal preparation, is a habit that was developed mostly by the body building community in order to accurately track your macronutrients. The basic idea behind meal prep is that each weekend, you manage your free time around cooking and preparing all of your meals for the upcoming week. While most meal preppers do their grocery shopping and cooking on Sundays, to keep their meals the freshest, you can choose to cook on a Saturday if that works better with your schedule. Meal preps each week uses one large grocery list of bulk ingredients to get all the supplies you need to make four dinners and four lunches of your choice. This means that you might have to do a bit of mental math quadrupling the serving size, but all you have to do is multiply each ingredient by four. Although you don't have to meal prep more than one meal with four portions each week, if you're already in the kitchen, you most likely have cooking time to work on something else.

Tracking Your Macronutrients

Wouldn't it be nice if you could have a full nutritional label for each of your home-cooked meals, just to make sure that your numbers are adding up in favor of weight loss? Oddly enough, tracking your macronutrients in order to calculate the nutritional value of each of your meals and portions is as easy as stepping on the scale. Not the scale in your bathroom, however. A food scales! If you've never had a good relationship with your weight and numbers, you might suddenly find that they aren't too bad after all. Food scales are used to measure, well, your food, but there's a slick system of online calculators and fitness applications for your smart phone that can take this number and turn it into magic. When your meal preps each week, keep track of your recipes diligently. Remember how you multiplied each of the ingredients on the list by four to create four servings? You're going to want to remember how much of each vegetable, fruit, grain, nut, and fat you cooked with. While you wait for your meal to finish cooking, find a large enough plastic container to fit all of your meals. Make sure it's clean and dry, and use the empty container to zero out your scale.

Counting Calories and Forming a Deficit

When it comes down to the technical science, there is one way and only one way to lose weight: by eating fewer calories in one day than your body requires to survive. Now, this doesn't mean that you can't lose weight for other reasons – be it water weight, as a result of stress, or simply working out harder. Although counting calories might not be the most fun way to lose weight, a calorie deficit is the only sure-fire way of guaranteeing that you reap all the weight loss benefits of the

Mediterranean diet for your efforts. Scientifically, you already know that the healthy rate of weight loss for the average adult is between one and two pounds per week. Get ready for a little bit more math, but it's nothing you can't handle in the name of a smaller waistline. One pound of fat equals around thirty-five hundred Calories, which means that your caloric deficit needs to account for that number, each week, without making too much of a dent on your regular nutrition. For most of us, we're used to eating between fifteen hundred and two thousand calories per day, which gives you a blessedly simply five hundred calorie deficit per day in order to reach your healthy weight loss goals. If you cut out exactly five hundred calories each day, you should be able to lose one pound of fat by the end of seven days. Granted, this estimate does take into account thirty minutes of daily exercise, but the results are still about the same when you rely on the scientific facts. If your age, height, weight, and sex predispose you to eat either more or less calories per day, you might want to consult with your doctor about the healthiest way for you to integrate a caloric deficit into your Mediterranean diet.

Goal Setting to Meet Your Achievements

On the subject of control, there are a few steps and activities that you should go through before you begin your Mediterranean diet just to make sure that you have clear and realistic goals in mind. Sitting down to set goals before embarking on a totally new diet routine will help you stay focused and committed during your Mediterranean diet. While a Mediterranean diet lifestyle certainly isn't as demanding as some of the crazy diet fads you see today, it can be a struggle to focus on eating natural fruits and vegetables that are more "salt of the Earth" foods than we're used to. You already know that when it comes to weight loss, you shouldn't expect to lose more than one to two pounds per week healthily while you're dieting. You are still welcome to set a weight loss goal with time in mind, but when it comes to the Mediterranean diet, you should set your goals for one month in the future.

Thanks, and best of luck.

CPSIA information can be obtained
at www.ICGtesting.com
Printed in the USA
LVHW081946170221
679362LV00002B/70